dementia
essentials

To my parents Jean and John Hall
and everyone touched by dementia.

dementia essentials

How to guide a loved one through Alzheimer's or Dementia and provide the best care

JAN HALL

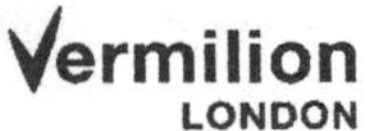

LONDON

5 7 9 10 8 6

Vermilion, an imprint of Ebury Publishing,
20 Vauxhall Bridge Road,
London SW1V 2SA

Vermilion is part of the Penguin Random House group of companies whose addresses can be found at global.penguinrandomhouse.com

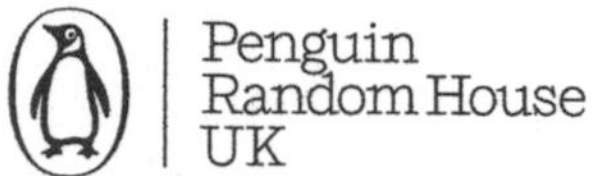

First published by Vermilion in 2013
www.penguin.co.uk

A CIP catalogue record for this book is available from the British Library

ISBN 9780091948160

Printed and bound in Great Britain by Clays Ltd, St Ives plc

Penguin Random House is committed to a sustainable future for our business, our readers and our planet. This book is made from Forest Stewardship Council® certified paper.

The author has generously donated the royalties from the sale of this book to Alzheimer's Society (registered Charity No. 296645) to help people with dementia and their carers. The opinions expressed in this book are the author's own and should not be regarded as the opinions of Alzheimer's Society.

CONTENTS

INTRODUCTION

Thank you for reading these words.

The inspiration behind this book came from loving families and friends who wanted to use their insights and experience of caring for their loved ones to try to reduce the burden for people encountering dementia for the first time. This aspires to be the book they would like to have been given when they first encountered this disease.

At the heart of *Dementia Essentials* are the experiences of people like you who realised that a loved one was living with dementia. They have struggled through often distressing decisions and heartbreak, and have bravely agreed to re-live some of the pain in order to help others who may find themselves in a similar situation. Their names, genders, relationships and personal circumstances have been changed to protect their privacy, allowing them to speak freely and honestly.

For me personally, I watched and tried to help my wonderful father do all that he could – and perhaps more than he should have done and she would have wanted – to look after the wife he so loved. He says caring for my mother was 'physically and mentally exhausting at a level I had never experienced before' but that he has now become 'a different person, more balanced and tolerant, and most of all happy that I did my best to care for my wife'.

For my part, my mother was my best friend and I hated losing our closeness as her Alzheimer's developed. Looking back, I was not kind enough to her in the early stages as I didn't fully understand what was happening to her and how much she needed me to put her needs first. It was easier to see what help she needed as she moved through the middle and especially the later stages. In many ways, because my father was totally devoted to caring for my mother, it was him as the carer who needed more of my care and, crucially, my understanding of how best to support them both.

There are so many things I wish I had known throughout my mother's illness and it is this regret that inspired me with this book to try to help other families embarking on a similar journey to mine. What you read here may make you cry. It may frighten you with a depiction of what dementia will bring. My abiding hope – and that of those who have so generously contributed to this project – is that you will be better prepared, learning from our mistakes and successes. It is our wish, as you live through this difficult and testing time, that the information, advice and shared experiences in this book will help you feel more supported and less alone.

Jan Hall

CHAPTER 1

talking about it

We just don't like talking about tricky personal subjects. Although the word 'taboo' had to be borrowed from Polynesian culture by Captain Cook, the idea of avoiding difficult topics as though they were unclean lies deep within the human psyche, and is perhaps at its most pronounced in British culture. Dementia introduces an unpleasant cocktail of taboos. Firstly, it's the beginning of the end, a long slide towards death – and we don't talk about death; secondly, it's a disease within the brain that interferes with people's perception of reality – and we don't talk about mental deficiencies; thirdly, it's a process that scrapes away layers of skills, memories and awareness, leading someone we love into delusion and confusion – and that's something we don't even want to think about.

But perhaps we should try to talk about these issues, bringing them out into the open and stripping them of their ability to get between us and the ones we love? Facing your fears and having that difficult conversation might remove years of anguish. And if there is a right time to confront these difficult topics it is probably sooner rather than later. How and when you approach this task will depend on your situation and your relationship with the person whom you fear might be in trouble.

Christa's husband had always been imaginative and eccentric, but she gradually realised that his increasingly wacky comments and gaps in his memories may have had a different cause. She watched his recall of recent events getting gradually worse, and discussed it with her children before broaching the subject with him.

'About six years ago, it got bad enough for me to have a conversation about his memory and whether he was coping as well as he used to. I was terrified of having this conversation because he was fiercely independent and I didn't want to offend him. But actually it went down very well. I think he had been worrying about it himself, because he seemed relieved that it was out in the open.'

Of course, that's not everybody's experience. The first person to notice the disturbing lapses of memory or serious confusion is almost always the person with dementia, who will often respond by retreating into private fears, defending their independence with vigour. Just by listening calmly, you can sense the distress behind the protective veneer of impatience that swats away other people's concerns.

When her father was more than an hour late getting back from a regular meeting with friends, Margaret was beginning to be anxious.

> **'He walked in, looking a bit flustered, but I didn't want to say anything to him because I knew that when I corrected him he would always get angry and respond that he was not going mad! So I stopped mentioning things. I had to, because he would get so upset.'**

Karen's approach was different, and she felt she had to challenge her mother directly when she didn't remember things, suggesting that perhaps there was something important underlying the increasingly common memory 'blips'.

> **'I said I thought she should go and have her memory tested. And she said there was nothing wrong with her, and would not even entertain a discussion about it. But as it became clearer that there was a problem, I became much more careful about how I approached it – because it was then obvious that there really was something wrong.'**

As her mother struggled to cover the gaps in her memory and retain her fading grasp on everyday life going on around her, Karen became conscious that the family was finding fault with her more and more often. Their days were peppered with comments such as 'But you just said that, Mum!', or 'I've just told you that, Mum!' and Karen began to sense the distress this might be causing.

'The more it dawned on me how real the problem actually was, the gentler I became with her. I was always worried about what was going on inside her head. What was she thinking? Was she terrified? And I just wanted to get in there and hug her or help her – and she wouldn't let me in.'

When you sense that someone you love might be developing a serious medical problem, of course you are going to be distressed. And if the person is unwilling to open up and discuss your concerns, then that is likely to increase your sense of frustration. But it may be no less frustrating for your loved one to be continually urged to deal with something that seems just too big for her to manage. So is it right to try and grasp the nettle? Should you go for confrontation?

'Most rational beings who are *not* in the middle of coping with a loved one who has dementia would say, "Of course you should tackle it head-on," because you want to discuss with them what you need to do and how you'll handle it together.'

There is obviously nothing but sense in that view. But life is very rarely that simple.

Every time Karen's mother went to see her doctor, he would apparently tell her she had dementia – and the whole family would know that the next few days were going to be hellish.

'My dad would always dread her going to the surgery because every time she'd be furious for the next few days and nothing would go right. Whenever she was forced into recognising what was actually happening to her, she would be appalling until she had forgotten what they had told her. I know that the professional view is that you should tell people and you should talk about it ... but I don't know if that is best.'

There is no 'one size fits all' answer, no simple rule to decide whether you should gently push someone whom you fear might be showing those first signs of dementia to talk about it and share her worries. The ideal solution is, of course, to have the conversation long before there is a cloud in the sky or any hint of a problem developing, because that is when the subject can be approached in an objective and totally unthreatening manner. Everyone can think about how best to approach the problem if it should arise, and agree on the best way to proceed, and then everyone can relax in the knowledge that you're all going to be on the same side with a 'disaster plan' at the ready. But, if you're reading this when that point has been passed, that advice is as unhelpful as somebody saying, 'Well, I wouldn't start from here ...' when you ask them for directions.

Adam's view is that the only way to overcome the taboo is to ignore it and speak out, approaching dementia in the same matter-of-fact way as you would deal with any other serious illness. He feels that hiding away the fear of suspected dementia is wrong, because you're losing the chance of starting treatment early and making arrangements before there is any serious deterioration.

'My father thought it was a real stigma and wanted to keep it a secret so he was horrified when I told my wife and her family. I explained to him that people need to know he has dementia, otherwise they will think he is being genuinely weird. You have to address it and be upfront about it. And by tackling it, you soon realise that you are not alone and can learn from other people's stories and experiences.'

Perhaps what Karen might have done was to state her fears calmly, as soon as she felt that her mother's difficulties were going beyond normal age-related issues, without making any demands on her.

'Maybe if I had known what I know now, I could have actually said to my mum: "Listen. I think you have got a problem, but I do understand that you don't want to talk about it. I know I'm scared and I imagine you're scared, but can we just discuss our fears? I think it would help us all just to state how we feel, but I don't want it to change how we are."'

Karen feels that her mother might have accepted the idea of just discussing the situation now and then, perhaps every few months or so, in order to feel they were containing and managing the problem.

'But I didn't even think to talk about it then. What I was actually saying was "I'm cross because I'm going to lose you". I was losing my best friend, my support. There she was, disappearing, and that was why I was so cross, because she was leaving me, and I could do nothing to help her.'

first suspicions

Dementia takes many different forms, and the first signs to be visible to others can vary enormously. Some people disguise the effects for years, and that concealment is one of the causes of the first hidden stages of dementia going undiagnosed or under-diagnosed in the earliest stages. Another reason is that many of the disparate symptoms can also be associated with other common conditions. The loss of mental agility and the confusion could be indicators of depression, stress, diabetes or thyroid problems, or they may be nothing more than the gradual effects of normal ageing.

'Most of what I noticed with my dad is in retrospect because it was hard to work out what was going on for a long time. He went missing on a walk for 10 hours which was quite scary, and there was a suspicion there was something wrong.

He came up with this story and said he'd been thrown off a bus and punched somebody.'

Although every month brings news of researchers making small advances in definitively spotting early signs of dementia, there is still no straightforward screening method that is cost-effective, practical and reliable enough for general use in making the earliest diagnosis. Until the understanding of the roots of dementia enables doctors to use something like a simple analysis of blood or saliva to detect indications of the physical changes in the brain, the first suspicions of dementia tend to be based on subjective observations of unusual behaviour – usually of forgetfulness or confusion, sometimes of behavioural changes. But the build-up of little incidents that may strike relatives or friends as unsettling can seem totally innocent to professionals who are trained to find hard evidence on which to base their opinions.

'We realised she was just doing slightly bizarre things like not remembering people, and completely losing track of time. She'd muddle up my brother with my dad, or tell me stories about events that happened during the war as though they had just taken place. They were quite subtle signs.'

We all have memory lapses, and forgetting the name of the woman who used to teach your daughter in primary school is not dementia. Our ability to store and recall data degrades as we get older, and it gets worse when we are stressed or tired. But people with dementia can seem to float in and out of different periods in their life, passing through the intervening decades like a ghost walking through a wall, before returning unsteadily to now. These occasional early time-slips can be hard to spot unless you know the person well or spend a fair amount of time in their company, but they can gradually build up into a disquiet that others may not share.

'It was me and her most of the time. My brother and sister had their own families and they couldn't believe what I was telling them. I was saying there was something wrong with Mum, but they said she was just lonely. But I knew there was something that was just not right.'

The first hints of confusion will often go unnoticed, or be put down to tiredness. Sometimes they are conspicuous enough to arouse comment and can provoke laughter and embarrassment, as people are oblivious of the struggle raging out of view against a reality that lurches in and out of focus.

'We noticed it when we went to the beach with her for a lovely day. On the way back we played a "Who am I?" guessing game, and she chose the same name – quite a distinctive name – three times in a row. She genuinely didn't remember that she'd already played that name several times. And we just laughed at her ...'

With some people, the first signs of disruption deep inside emerge in unexpected ways. Character traits that have always been present may become more evident or exaggerated, and particular facets of personality may appear to be intensified. Small differences of opinion can develop into unfamiliar battlegrounds, as people with dementia struggle to win arguments, perhaps to conceal a growing sense that they may be losing control.

Linda feels that dementia began to skew certain parts of her mother's character.

'She had always been quite stubborn, but when the dementia started it became much more difficult to deal with her because she would be absolutely certain that she was correct. We would end up having quite large rows over silly things like the colour of my trousers or whether a picture in her house was straight. I started thinking, "What the hell's the matter with this woman?"'

One behavioural change that is often associated with the early days of dementia is depression. Many of the symptoms – apathy, indifference, negative introspection, a fear of new challenges, poor memory performance – can be common to both.

James was initially worried by his mother's increasing listlessness, and a general loss of interest in the life that was going on around her.

'Mum had never been a depressed person, but she just started to get very down and didn't want to

go and do things – she always made excuses. I eventually took her to the doctor to try and get to the bottom of it, and he diagnosed depression.'

It's not unusual for GPs to prescribe antidepressants as a first measure, if only to rule out depression as the origin of the apathy before delving deeper to see if the cause may lie elsewhere. It's easy to understand that being conscious of a gradual loss of cognitive abilities and self-confidence could drag someone into a negative spiral of rumination, but research also suggests that people with a history of depression may be more likely to develop dementia in later years.

Susan's mother had always felt that life had been harsh to her, and this bitterness gave way to depression and a joyless inertia as she grew older. She would stay in bed until lunchtime, and then often wander aimlessly around a shopping centre for most of the day, before returning home to watch television until she went to bed.

'And that was her rhythm. Unless somebody asked her to do something, nothing happened to her. She rarely generated any interest or excitement for herself, and would avoid going to places where there were strangers – like a library, a film, a café or an evening class. So she never bumped into people the way that most of us do. She became terrifically isolated, virtually insulated from any interactions with others.'

Some individuals simply recoil from a world that seems to dance mockingly before their eyes. Unable or unwilling to share the inner fears that their memory and powers of reasoning are declining, they may struggle to carry on with their usual habits until it all becomes too much to cope with.

Brenda remembers how concerned she was one day when her husband was several hours late coming home from a local shopping trip.

> 'When he finally got home, he seemed very unsettled. I looked in his coat pockets later and found loads of bus tickets, even though he had a bus pass. He'd obviously been on quite a few buses before he managed to get home. And then I noticed that he stopped wanting to go to church, or wanting to go to the top of the road, even just to pick up milk or something.'

Denise had got used to her husband being slightly vague and even seeming to get lost in places he knew quite well. And then one day he drove the wrong way down the motorway.

> 'The consultant told me that a high proportion of people with dementia have these visuo-spatial problems of perception. They can see okay, but the brain misinterprets what they are seeing – and that is the root of some strange behaviours, like confusing left and right.'

When someone fears that their mind may be deserting them, it's only natural to feel like drawing the wagons into a circle to keep out a hostile future. But health professionals and people who have been through the experience of caring for a loved one all agree that early diagnosis is vitally important. Try to persuade anyone who is worried about memory lapses and the possibility of dementia to make an appointment with the GP – people who go to the doctor may be sent home with the good news that their fears were unfounded. The worst that can happen if the problem is confirmed is that they are given the chance to fight back by planning the best possible future for them and their loved ones, and by starting treatment that may slow the progress of the dementia.

what you can do

The shock of learning that a family member or friend is living with dementia can be truly devastating. But take a good deep breath, because the diagnosis is not the end, but just the beginning. Throw away right now the idea of giving up, of losing all hope, because whoever is being consumed by dementia – parent, spouse, lover or friend – has never needed your love and support as acutely as they do now.

Whether or not you are going to be the main carer, take comfort from knowing that supportive family and friends working together can help enormously in easing the distress of a person with dementia – and may even be able to slow the decline by ensuring that medical intervention is sought as early as possible. Every stage of this cruel disease can be alleviated in some way by understanding the pathology of dementia, how it is likely to develop and how people might respond to the slow destruction of brain cells. And you can start by ensuring that you – and they – are prepared for what lies ahead.

so where should you start?

Many of the symptoms in the early stages of dementia only become apparent with hindsight, as others look back to wonder when it all started. Even before you have any worries about someone's memory or general cognitive abilities, it's important to foster active independence, while keeping an eye on things and quietly planning ahead. Doing whatever you can to encourage older people to enjoy an active and stimulated life is a big step towards fending off the threat of dementia; and emphasising the benefits of staying fit and heart-healthy will also help enormously.

If you feel that somebody may be moving beyond normal age-related confusion, the first step is to try to discuss it in a gentle and unthreatening way. Give reassurance that early action is better than dodging unspoken concerns and then worrying corrosively in secret. Encourage your loved one to explore the possible causes of any confusion with the GP. Work hard to work together, but work gently, emphasising the 'we' and offering to find out together what can be done.

Your next action will depend on the GP's view of the situation. If there is no sign of dementia, carry on as above, keep matters under review and use the relief everyone will feel as a pretext to start 'what if' discussions about the future. If there are signs of dementia, or even a full diagnosis, then it is time to take serious formal steps to safeguard the future and to avoid later complications. Those who have been through the caring process recommend that you should immediately look into drawing up a Power of Attorney (see pages 67–70), so that the best decisions can be taken. Discuss what medication is available, and push for early action. Start to share the news and build up the network of friends and family who will support the person with dementia in whatever way they can – with love, with practical help or with companionship.

The GP should refer the person with dementia to a psychiatrist specialising in dementia care and, in many places but not everywhere, to a 'memory clinic'. Accepting these referrals is vital because these experts will help find the most suitable drugs, ensure help is forthcoming from social-care departments and also support carers. Some of these memory clinics may offer the chance to help in research on the effectiveness of new treatments.

Although the natural caring instinct may be to help someone with dementia in any way possible, experts suggest that encouraging social activity and independence in the early stages is in fact more useful, as this will provide stimulation and avoid undermining self-confidence.

The middle stages are a time of growing upheaval for people with dementia. This may be reflected in aggression, probably due to frustration at their shrinking abilities and bewilderment as the world appears to hamper their every move. It can also reveal itself in a stifling lack of self-belief as they cling to their carers, showing great distress in their absence. But those around the person with dementia can make a huge difference in how the disease progresses. Care that is given with calm reassurance is the best sort of nurturing care, and you can channel your frustrations into giving you the energy and steely determination to get the most out of local authority care services and the other official bodies you will need to deal with.

This is the time to build relationships with the social-care providers and with the many organisations that can offer help and support to carers and to people with dementia. Keep an open mind on the best options for care as circumstances change, and try to prepare for the future. You will not know the timescale of the decline, but you do know how your loved one's capabilities and awareness will deteriorate and you will want to have the next steps prepared before they are suddenly needed.

By the final stages, dementia may appear to carry people far beyond communication with those around them, but the person you love is still in there and can still draw comfort from – and sometimes respond to – gentle affection or soothing voices, and many find solace in music or a simple loving touch.

However, as Neville explained, there is a lot to learn and do before you get to those end stages.

'At the start I was incredibly naïve and thought the system would look after my wife – and I thought our doctor would know exactly what to do. If I was starting again, I would try to read and learn about the whole subject. You have to be prepared to push to get help at most steps along the way.'

CHAPTER 2

dementia explained

what is dementia?

Dementia is not a single disease with a single cause, but a collection of symptoms characterised by the progressive loss of cognitive abilities. This deterioration within the brain affects memory, understanding, behaviour, judgement and ultimately the ability to perform the simple tasks of everyday life. People whose decline has led to a diagnosis of dementia before the age of 65 are said to have early-onset dementia, and they may represent up to 5 per cent of the UK's total cases of dementia; but the vast majority of people with dementia are diagnosed after the age of 65 and this is referred to as late-onset dementia.

Although it used to be regarded as just a normal inescapable part of ageing, late-onset dementia is, in fact, a chronic condition in which the overall rate and pattern of decline can vary considerably between individual patients, and the brain functions degenerate at different speeds in different forms of the condition.

So what are the various types of dementia?

Alzheimer's disease (named after the German scientist who first described the symptoms over a century ago) is the most common cause of late-onset dementia, responsible for around 60–70 per cent of all cases. The disease interferes with the proper healthy functioning of parts of the brain, preventing nerve cells (neurons) within the brain from communicating with and responding to other brain cells, and the cells affected eventually die. Brain scans of people with advanced Alzheimer's show extensive shrinkage in specific areas of the brain, and the damage is first visible in parts that are connected with memory functions, which is why serious memory blips are often the first detected symptoms of Alzheimer's disease.

It is not yet clear exactly how the disease works, but it is associated with two strange structures that appear in microscopic form inside ageing brains: *amyloid plaques* and *neurofibrillary tangles*. The plaques are chiefly made up of a protein fragment called beta-amyloid, which in certain circumstances clumps together to form these insoluble plaques. The tangles within brain cells are mainly formed from another proteins called tau, the normal role of which is to stabilise vital parts of the cell structure. In Alzheimer's disease this tau separates and forms abnormal twisted tangles with other tau filaments, which disrupts the ability of one neuron to transmit messages and nutrients to other neurons.

Scientific researchers are working hard to discover more about the details and sequence of events leading to the Alzheimer's damage. For example, we do not know whether the plaques and tangles are a cause of the disease or a product of the disease, and both abnormal structures have been found in the brains of people without dementia symptoms.

In the second most common form of late-onset dementia – called *vascular dementia* – damage to the brain cells is caused by a break in the flow of blood to the brain, which starves areas of the brain of the oxygen they need, causing the death of brain cells from lack of nutrition. Vascular dementia can be caused by a single major stroke, in which case the symptoms are likely to be suddenly evident, but it is more often the outcome of a series of mini-strokes, which you may hear GPs or medical staff describe as *transient ischemic attacks*, or TIAs. In the case of these repeated mini-strokes, the episodic nature of the interruptions to the supply of oxygen is typically mirrored in a stepped decline in abilities, compared to the more gradual degeneration typical of Alzheimer's disease, but this can depend on the number and intensity of the TIAs and how the consequent decline is handled or hidden.

'He had these mini-strokes, and it all got dealt with fine, but I think that was when he mentally started deteriorating. When our daughter came back from abroad, she noticed that he had got much worse. I was finding him more difficult really, rather than understanding there was a medical reason.'

Vascular dementia may also result from deterioration of the blood vessels leading to or inside the brain. If fatty deposits build up inside these tiny tubes, which feed oxygen and nutrients to brain cells, they can harden and gradually 'fur up' inside, like a kettle or water pipes in areas with 'hard' water. Among the known risk factors for this atherosclerosis are diabetes, lack of exercise and obesity.

Dementia with Lewy bodies is another form of the illness, the name describing tiny protein deposits first found in the brains of people with Parkinson's disease by scientist Frederick Lewy a century ago. As awareness of dementia grew, researchers noted the presence of the same harmful protein deposits in the brains of people with the condition. It is still an under-diagnosed form of dementia, partly because it shares many symptoms with Alzheimer's (such as the decline in cognitive functions) and Parkinson's (deterioration in motor control), and is frequently confused with both diseases. The first signs displayed by people with this dementia type may be either Parkinson's-like or Alzheimer's-like, but both sets of symptoms will emerge as the disease progresses. This form of dementia is also often characterised by powerful hallucinations, fluctuating levels of cognitive ability and sleep disorders.

Fronto-temporal dementia is the result of shrinkage of tissue in the frontal lobes (situated, unsurprisingly, at the front of the brain, above the eyes) and temporal lobes (above and behind the ears) of the brain. These areas control 'executive functions', including the ability to plan and think things through and the capacity to act appropriately in social contexts, and also manage speech and language. People with this form of dementia are prone to losing some or all inhibitions and acting impulsively, and their self-restraint and awareness of how to behave around other people can dissolve completely. Some people with fronto-temporal dementia also experience muscular and movement disorders, such as shakiness, spasms or problems with balance.

However, cases of dementia can often show symptoms of more than one of these disease types, and it is not uncommon for people to be diagnosed with a combination of Alzheimer's disease and vascular dementia, or Alzheimer's and one of the less common variants.

Alcohol-related dementia has been described as the silent epidemic, because most people are unaware that the decline in cognitive functions seen in dementia can also be triggered by the persistent over-consumption of alcohol. The long-term misuse of alcohol interferes with the body's ability to use or store vitamins, particularly vitamin B1, which affects the functioning of the nervous system and the brain, leading to memory loss and personality changes. Unlike other forms of dementia, if caught soon enough, alcohol-related dementia can be reversed: a quarter of people with alcohol-related dementia recover completely, but another quarter are permanently damaged. Drinking that falls short of alcohol abuse but is habitually above the recommended levels is said to be a contributory factor in between 20 and 25 per cent of all dementia cases, and there are fears that a growing number of young people will be affected.

Less common diseases that may also lead to dementia include Parkinson's and Huntington's, HIV and AIDS,

Creutzfeldt-Jakob disease, multiple sclerosis and motor neurone disease.

Although researchers are gradually uncovering new details of how dementia is caused, there is currently no cure. The medical treatments that are available work only on the symptoms, and – if given early enough – may delay cognitive decline, so that people with dementia can stave off the more dependent later stages of the condition.

'All the research seems to say that the earlier you take the drugs, the better. So if people have any sense of entering the early stages of dementia, the sooner they can start taking the drugs, the longer they will have. There's actually a medical urgency to get people to tackle it now.'

The main drugs prescribed for treating Alzheimer's disease are acetylcholinesterase inhibitors (ACEIs, for short). They work by slowing down the effects of a natural enzyme – acetylcholinesterase – which breaks down a substance called acetylcholine. The brains of people with Alzheimer's disease show significantly lower levels of this chemical, an important neurotransmitter that has a key role in forming and processing short-term memories. So the effect of the ACEIs is to boost the level of acetylcholine in the brain cells, by reducing the rate at which the enzyme breaks it down.

The three ACEI drugs approved for use in the UK are donepezil (commonly known by the brand name Aricept), rivastigmine (common brand name Exelon) and galantamine (common brand name Reminyl), and these last two also impact on other useful neurotransmitters. All three drugs are now recommended for use by people with mild or moderate dementia. They are usually prescribed by a specialist and are subject to regular review to ensure that they are having a positive effect on symptoms. A specialist committee asked to appraise the three ACEI drugs by the National Institute for Health and Clinical Excellence (NICE) decided that there was not enough evidence to differentiate between them in terms of their clinical effectiveness.

Some side effects, such as nausea, headaches and diarrhoea, are not uncommon and specialists considering which drug to prescribe will need to take into account general health issues and any history of heart, kidney or liver problems.

'The specialist said get her on Aricept quickly if you want to get any benefit from it. The thing about Aricept is that it keeps you level for a lot longer, and then when you drop off you drop off fast. It doesn't give you a lot more life, but the brain lasts longer in its current state.'

A fourth drug – memantine (common brand name Ebixa) – works by tempering the harmful action of another neurotransmitter – glutamate – while allowing it to continue carrying out its 'good' role related to learning and memory functions. It has been used with positive outcomes on patients in the later stages of Alzheimer's disease, and has had success in addressing agitation and aggression. There is some clinical evidence that a combination of memantine and an ACEI – most commonly donepezil – can have a greater effect than the ACEI drug administered on its own.

Whichever drug or drugs the specialist prescribes, it can be a good idea to keep a diary of any side effects (such as nausea or dizziness) that the person with dementia experiences. The more feedback you can give, the more chance you have of ensuring that the right medication is prescribed – and the only way to keep track when so much else is going on is to write things down. In the later stages, when the person with dementia has lost most cognitive functions, treatment with these drugs is usually discontinued.

The choice of medication to relieve symptoms of the other forms of dementia is less clear-cut. Although some research suggests that ACEIs may improve cognition in the early stages of vascular dementia, more attention is focused on measures to lower the risk of further TIAs, such as lowering blood pressure and cholesterol levels, and controlling diabetes and heart disease. For fronto-temporal dementia, there is no recommended medication to control the disease's progress, although doctors may suggest measures to tackle symptoms or behavioural issues. People diagnosed as having dementia with Lewy bodies may be given treatment for the symptoms, but there is a tendency for drugs that alleviate one of the groups of symptoms (physical issues, such as tremors and muscle movements, or psychiatric issues e.g. behavioural changes) to enhance the other type of symptom. In some cases prescription of ACEI drugs may give relief to people with this form of dementia.

People with dementia may also sometimes be prescribed specific medicines to control agitation or aggression. Use of these antipsychotic drugs has been the target of campaigns, and guidelines have been drawn up to limit the frequency with which they are prescribed. Institutions, such as care homes and hospitals, are under pressure to look for alternative non-pharmacological remedies to reduce aggression or agitation in people with dementia – behavioural therapies, stimulating activities or simple pain relief are a few of the measures that can address the causes behind 'troublesome' behaviours.

A major review of the role of antipsychotic drugs in dementia care emphasised that reducing the over-prescribing of antipsychotic drugs to people with dementia is now a national requirement, and they should normally be used only in the most serious cases when other measures have been tried and failed.

'Some people do benefit from these drugs but many experience potentially serious adverse effects, including increased mortality, and these can manifest with relatively short-term use. Antipsychotic drugs produce a range of complications that increase the rate of admission to hospital.'

Hopes are still very much alive that the energetic research work in labs around the world can produce more effective treatments for all forms of dementia, and ultimately ways of preventing the various diseases from causing degeneration in brain tissue. The breakthrough may come from existing medicines for other diseases (a drug aimed at diabetes has been shown to reverse memory decline in laboratory experiments), from targeting other brain cells (new research suggests that suppressing the actions of certain astrocyte cells may reduce levels of toxic amyloid in the brain) or from a completely new angle as yet undiscovered.

you are not alone

The words 'dementia' and 'success' do not sit comfortably together in the same sentence. Yet the increase in the numbers of people with dementia that we can see around us – and the scary projections of further growth, which are slowly heaving the machinery of change into action – is connected to the success in tackling other illnesses and in prolonging the average lifespan.

The primary risk factor for developing dementia is age. The longer we live, the higher the likelihood that we will experience brain decay and all that comes with it. And humans are surviving longer than ever before. The weight of the Department for Work and Pensions has been placed behind a prediction that one in four children alive today in the UK can expect to receive a telegram (or the digital equivalent) from the monarch in due course.

The 20th century, in Britain as elsewhere, was a time of enormous changes in people's lives and these were matched by transformations in how and when people died. In 1880

– the year when the light bulb was first patented – infectious and parasitic diseases were responsible for a third of all deaths in the UK, but by 1997 this figure had been halved. Advances in scientific understanding and techniques, together with the social improvements brought about by growing affluence (such as better sanitation, hygiene and nutrition), slashed mortality from infectious diseases. The 440 sad UK deaths from tuberculosis in 1997, for example, are dwarfed by the approximately 80,000 people who were killed by the same disease in 1880. And whereas the official figures for 1911 show that nearly two-thirds of British people died without ever reaching their 60th birthday, by the last decade of the century just 12 per cent suffered similarly 'premature' deaths.

One result of the fact that we are generally living longer – coupled with a drop in birth rates – is that the average age of the population is sharply increasing. The familiar pyramid shape of the horizontal bar chart of age groups – the youngest age groups forming the largest section at the bottom, rising to the dwindling older groups at the top – has been remodelled into something more like a wobbly Jenga tower of wooden blocks. These changes have led prominent political economist Francis Fukuyama to speculate on whether this 'geriatric revolution' will eventually cause society to resemble 'a giant nursing home'.

At the turn of the millennium, the Population Division of the United Nations Secretariat estimated that the world population of over-60s was 605 million, and predicted that by the middle of this century that figure would reach two billion.

For the first time in history, the number of older people (those aged over 60) will match the number of children (aged up to 14). So by 2050 the current percentage of older people in the population – 10 per cent of the world population, but 20 per cent in the more developed regions, and 8 per cent in the less developed regions – will have more than doubled overall to 22 per cent of the world population (that's 33 per cent and 21 per cent respectively in the more developed and less developed regions).

The fastest-growing segment of that ageing population – a category numbered in 2000 at some 70 million people around the world, with twice as many women as men – is those aged 80 years or more. UN forecasts predict that by the year 2050 this group of the 'oldest old' will be five times larger than it was in 2000; and in the more developed regions nearly 10 per cent of the population will be in that 'oldest old' age group, where between one in five and one in six people will have a form of dementia.

But why does this happen? Is the deterioration of the brain wiring just 'unplanned obsolescence', the breakdown of parts that simply need replacing? Scientists are still trying to understand what is happening at the molecular level as we age, and there is a global push to sift through data on all age-related conditions in the hope of finding a common factor that would explain the molecular processes that make the ageing brain more susceptible to disease. Individual pieces of the jigsaw are becoming clearer, and occasionally fitting together, but the overall picture is still beyond our grasp.

what is memory?

It's never easy to give any substance to large numbers. If I have to picture a hundred objects, I can usually manage to conjure up in my mind an ordered grid of 10 rows of 10 blobs. If I am being asked to imagine a thousand somethings, I can just about 'zoom out' to encompass 10 of those 10 x 10 grids, in the style of an aerial view of a formation of Roman soldiers. To visualise 70,000, I mentally mingle with the crowd in an almost full Millennium Stadium. But beyond that, it's a struggle.

So what is the best way of picturing just how complicated the human brain is? Even though research scientists have recently lowered their estimate of the number of neurons to be found in an average human brain from the suspiciously tidy figure of 100 billion, they reckon that we still have at least 86 billion of these tiny impulse-transmitting cells in our brains. Can you picture 86 billion? Is that a bigger number than measuring the height of Mount Everest in millimetres? No, Everest is a paltry nine million millimetres high, and we have 10,000 times as many neurons as that. How about the number of seconds in a lengthy lifespan of 80 years? No, that's only 2.5 billion, and you would need 34 times that number to match our neuron count. Try to imagine the total number of people who have ever lived on this planet, from the earliest humans thousands of years ago up until the present day, and that's much closer to the number of neurons in an average brain. Or if technology is more your thing, count the number of tweets that have been sent since the micro-messaging service Twitter began and you will find there are roughly two tweets for each neuron (although there is no evidence that most tweets require any neurons at all).

If you're still with me, now is the time to take a deep breath. Those neurons transmit information around the brain at speeds of up to 100 metres per second, and they spread their messages through multiple connections, sparking the data by chemical transmission across smaller-than-microscopic gaps called synapses. The estimates of the number of synapses between your ears are simply stunning: within the cerebral cortex alone (that's the outer, visible part of the brain, which makes up 70 per cent of its volume and is responsible for the so-called higher functions – thought, memory, awareness and action among them) it has been calculated that there are between 60 and 240 trillion synapses. So you may have nearly a thousand times more synapses in your 1.3 kilograms of grey brain cells than there are stars in the whole of the 100,000-light-year-wide Milky Way.

It can be useful to keep those extraordinary statistics in mind if you ever find yourself looking at a real brain in a laboratory. The smallish lump of grimly grey tissue is singularly unimpressive, rather like a squidgy giant walnut. It is not difficult to understand why even someone as clever as Aristotle, ignoring the earlier views of Plato and Hippocrates, looked at the brain and concluded that it was simply a convoluted maze of tubes to cool the blood – presumably to prevent 'hot-headedness' – while the heart was clearly controlling all the body's processes and was the centre of the emotions, sensations and movements of the body.

So how does the brain store memories? Well, although we are only at the stage of theorising how it is done, we have a far more sophisticated model than the Ancient Greek suggestion that the process of retaining thoughts and memories was like making impressions in soft wax. Psychologists define memory as the ability to store and retrieve information, and in simple terms they split the process of forming memories into three distinct phases or types of memory: sensory memory, which receives input from any of the five senses, and lasts a second or two at most; short-term memory, where a limited number of objects or facts are held for a short time, perhaps around 20 seconds, before being either lost or passed on; and long-term memory, where everything you wish to remember – and things you might rather forget – accumulate and can persist for a lifetime.

In order to look at the memory mechanisms in a little more depth, you can think of short-term memory as like a rough notepad for jotting down facts you need at hand, or like the RAM (random access memory) in your computer that holds what you are working on before it is stored (or saved). Our knowledge of how the memory works has developed through studying people who have suffered damage to certain parts of the brain, where memories are encoded or stored. Psychologists believe that this 'working memory' contains different elements that capture stimuli from different sources – visual data, spoken or written language – and are controlled by a 'central executive' function at the front of the brain (the prefrontal cortex). This regulates how much of the important stuff is sent into long-term memory storage.

At its best, memory is an extraordinary and elastic function. A super-champion of memory has memorised the order of the 52 cards in a shuffled pack in 100 seconds. Contrast that staggering feat with the flickering frailty of our everyday memory failings, as we reach the top of the stairs without a clue about what urgent desire sent us up there. Our memories have been shown to be affected by our mood, to be disrupted by the weather conditions, and they can be – as in the cases of eye-witnesses of significant events who disagree on the most fundamental details of what happened – peculiarly unreliable and open to suggestion and manipulation. Researchers have demonstrated that our memories may work better when we are walking at a decent speed than when we are stationary, that stress affects our ability to create new memories and that the simple act of walking through a doorway (even if you are walking at a decent speed!) can diminish our chances of remembering what we were doing in the room we just left.

When the Alzheimer's form of dementia causes the death of brain cells and stifles the connections that carry data through the brain, it targets parts of the cerebral cortex that are involved in planning and memory functions. It appears to wreak most havoc in the hippocampus, a tiny area in the temporal lobe of the brain that is believed to play a major part in the creation of new memories by transferring the fickle contents of working memory (or short-term memory) to more stable storage in long-term memory, and which also plays a role in spatial awareness.

It's so easy to think of memory loss as simply forgetting where you put your glasses, or losing track of people's names at a party. But when something like dementia sweeps away the recollection of whole chunks of a life, the damage goes far, far deeper than that. We all secretly want to be 'unforgettable' to people we meet, and we praise holidays, meals or occasions as 'memorable'. To be 'forgotten' implies sadness and dusty rejection. 'How would you like to be remembered?' is a well-worn question that every interviewer will expect celebrities to answer in an interesting way when ideas run short.

The patchwork quilt of individual memories, assembled over a lifetime, is the timeline that explains 'the you-ness of you'. It traces your personal evolution, and illustrates how you have become what you are, and why you are where you are. And as pathways within someone's brain are blocked by the physical effects of dementia, the framework of that person's life begins to give way, and the whole structure can collapse, shutting out parts of that life, knocking other phases out of sequence and making individual segments of his or her own history janglingly foreign to the person who lived them.

So if people in mid-stage dementia 'lose' the memories of their children growing up and leaving home, then they can only conclude that those strange layabouts who claim to be their offspring must be impostors and frauds. And if the disruption of moving the family out of the noisy city into the peace of the countryside has been erased from their life story, then every glimpse of green meadows through the window will surely convince them that they've been kidnapped and must do everything possible to escape.

Once people with dementia have 'lost' some of those memories, their actual experiences of 'today' may become inexplicable to them, or just one of a range of possible outcomes, none of which is more convincingly real than any other.

Sam's mother had been becoming increasingly vague for years, but he was brought up short one day when she started imagining that a relative who had died years earlier was going to call in and visit her.

> **'When I asked her how her day had gone, she said she had been sitting there all day waiting for her sister to come over and she still hadn't come. Of course, I knew there was something wrong then, because her sister had been dead for 10 years. But when I reminded her of that, she got really upset and cried, and said, "Don't you dare say things like that!" She insisted that she was still at the wedding and would be coming along soon.'**

Our memories differentiate us from others. In some sense, our memories define us, and that may be why we defend them with such passion. All our experiences, all those treasured feelings that bind us to places and to people, the shared moments that cement our relationships ... these are what flutter out of our grasp as dementia erodes the foundations of who we are. Memories of the best times of our lives warm and nourish us, and the converse is also true: memories of traumas and negative experiences are also stored, whether we like it or not. But even when the actual memory of events and experiences is turned to dust by dementia, the feelings linger like a half-remembered dream, beyond the reach of conscious thought. These may be negatives, like guilt, fear or loss, or more positive emotions, such as the pleasure created by your last visit to a friend in need, which you may see resurfacing in a welcoming smile, even though the accompanying details of what you did together may be lost for ever.

Writing 200 years ago in her novel *Mansfield Park*, Jane Austen allowed one of her characters to wax lyrical on the frustrating unpredictability of our memories.

> *If any one faculty of our nature may be called more wonderful than the rest, I do think it is memory. There seems something more speakingly incomprehensible in the powers, the failures, the inequalities of memory, than in any other of our intelligences. The memory is sometimes so retentive, so serviceable, so obedient; at others, so bewildered and so weak; and at others again, so tyrannic, so beyond control! We are, to be sure, a miracle every way; but our powers of recollecting and of forgetting do seem peculiarly past finding out.*

research shows ...

You wouldn't slap a contributor to scientific research, would you? Even one who continually buzzes around your fruit bowl, lured by the smell of ripe bananas? So let's have a bit of respect for little *Drosophila melanogaster*, better known (and cursed!) as the humble fruit fly, and celebrated as an unwitting partner in the research that won the 1995 Nobel Prize in Medicine.

If you read through a list of research projects, you will find fruit flies in every corner, but why do scientists study these little pests in such detail? The short answer is quite long. Firstly, their structure is simple enough to be relatively easy to work on and yet they are sufficiently complex to be worth studying. Secondly, they have a short lifecycle, so quickly show the effects of whatever is tried out on them. And thirdly, there is a remarkable 60 per cent similarity between their genetic make-up and that of humans, which makes them very special tools in the quest to uncover the origins of human development and diseases. They also have unexpected similarities to humans that make them intriguingly relevant as a testing partner: social isolation has been shown to shorten their lifespan, they sleep deeply at night in a favourite sleeping position and when fed alcohol, they become hyperactive and then pass out. Does any of that sound familiar?

In the 100 years since they were first put under a microscope, scientists have discovered all about the little fly's genetic structure and mapped all 13,600 of its little genes. And as human-disease genes can often be matched to fruit fly genes, working on the flies allows scientists to carry out experiments that would be impossible – not to mention unethical – on humans, and would in any case produce workable data only after several human generations. The results of those experiments impact directly on the understanding of diseases, of memory processes and even of ageing itself. Fruit flies have, for example, recently been part of some exciting research into a tiny micro-RNA regulator molecule that is linked with the ageing process. When flies are born without this regulator, they age much more quickly, and the opposite is also true: when they are given extra doses, their median lifespan is extended.

So what has medical research – using fruit flies or larger volunteers – found that you can use to protect yourself against dementia? Take the bad news first: scientists have not yet found a 'smoking gun', the single habit or practice with a direct causal link to dementia, comparable to the breakthrough recognition in the 1950s of the relationship between smoking and lung cancer. Bear in mind that no single study is likely to yield a perfect simple mantra that will ward off dementia. But the good news is that experts believe there are 'modifiable risk factors' – lifestyle changes or medical interventions that would reduce an individual's risk of developing dementia. The risk factors for vascular dementia are well documented – including obesity, high blood pressure, irregular heartbeat, raised cholesterol levels – and it seems that they may be more generally related to other forms of dementia as well. The current wisdom on the sensible precautions you might wish to take could be broadly summed up in the thought that what's 'good for your heart' also appears to be 'good for your brain'. And, reduced to a bumper sticker, that would read 'moderation is good': moderation in what you eat, and moderation in everything.

EAT WELL: Advice on maintaining a heart-healthy lifestyle is fairly mainstream nowadays, and any diet that emphasises fresh fruit and vegetables is certainly one that a cardiologist would recommend. Highlighted in various studies are the benefits of food that is rich in omega-3 fatty acids – such as fish and nuts (salmon and walnuts get particular praise). Approach your meals with an eye for colour: green vegetables are good, but purple fruits (such as blueberries) have been singled out in research as particularly beneficial. You'd do well to avoid excess consumption of carbohydrates and sugar: tracking over a thousand elderly people for four years revealed that those with the highest carbohydrate intake were nearly twice as likely to develop mild cognitive impairment (MCI – which can lead to symptoms of dementia) as participants with the lowest portions of carbohydrate on their plates. Those eating food with the highest levels of sugar showed a 50 per cent increase in the risk of developing MCI, but those on diets highest in fat saw a 42 per cent reduction in that risk.

SLEEP WELL: See 'Sleep' on pages 148–54.

LOSE WEIGHT: Keeping trim in your 30s, 40s and 50s could reduce the risk of dementia later in life. Confirming earlier data, a Swedish study found that people classed as overweight or obese in middle age had an 80 per cent higher risk of developing dementia, even when other contributory factors – such as vascular disease and diabetes – were taken into account. Yes, 80 (not 8) per cent!

AVOID STRESS: Lack of sleep and stress may of course be connected, but stress really slows us down. It can prevent the working memory from retaining information required for tasks in hand, exciting extra action in neurons in the prefrontal cortex but actually reducing their focus. Acute stress has been shown to trigger the release of hormones in the hippocampus, which interfere with the brain's collection and storage of memories. Research suggests that fitter people are more capable of managing stress than those who do not get enough exercise. A good walk for half an hour three times a week can make a real improvement in stress levels.

KEEP MOVING: Physical activity stimulates both the body and the brain, and regular exercise at a moderate level for 20 to 30 minutes can make an enormous difference to your health, cutting the risks of cardiovascular disease and strokes. That doesn't mean you have to throw money at a gym membership – walking briskly and dusting off your bicycle can make a big contribution. If you are not used to exercise, then start off gently, and rejoice in the knowledge that exercise can also help lower your blood pressure, reduce your risk of developing diabetes, improve your cholesterol levels, boost your self-esteem, cut levels of anxiety and depression, lift your mood by releasing endorphins, help you sleep better ... it's a wonder that nobody has thought of charging you for a half-hour's walk in the park!

KEEP HAPPY: See 'Change your mind' on pages 175–79.

REDUCE BLOOD PRESSURE: High blood pressure in early middle age has been shown to cause damage to the brain, making the brains of younger people 'age' more quickly and shrink – MRI scans showed that the brains of subjects with high blood pressure had shrunk by an average of 9 per cent, compared to the brains of people with normal blood pressure. Watch what you eat: try more foods such as oats, bananas, lean meat and low-fat dairy products, and less saturated fat, salt and added sugar. Lose weight if you are overweight, take more exercise and be prepared to cut down on excessive alcohol consumption.

DIABETES: Research is uncovering more suggestions of links between diabetes and Alzheimer's disease, including evidence that higher levels of two of the established pointers towards the presence of Alzheimer's – the beta-amyloid and tau proteins that seem to malfunction to form the plaques and tangles in brain cells – are found in the brains of animals with diabetes. The brains of people with diabetes in middle age have been shown to shrink faster, especially in the hippocampus – an area associated with memory function. If enough of these risk factors sound like you or someone you know – overweight, urinating frequently at night, constantly thirsty, with a history of diabetes in the family – then ask your GP to test for diabetes. It can sneak up gradually, but the good news is that it can be controlled.

HAVE A CUP: It's probably not the reason you made that delicious cup of coffee, but there's something in there that seems to increase levels of granulocyte colony stimulating factor (GCSF) in our blood. Neuroscientists don't yet know exactly how or why it happens (and it won't happen in your cup of decaf, because there's some interaction with the caffeine content), but it's a potential health benefit because doses of

GCSF have been shown to improve memory in lab experiments by boosting the production of new brain cells – and people with Alzheimer's disease have unusually low GCSF levels.

DON'T CORK IT: Would sir or madam like a glass of resveratrol? There is some evidence that this compound, found in wine and chocolate, may slow the deterioration of memory functions in people with Alzheimer's disease. It is also found in less exciting foods, such as grapes, tomatoes and peanuts. Red wine has much higher levels than white wine, but experts maintain that more research is needed before they recommend that everyone should uncork. And moderation is the watchword: moderate drinkers may see benefits – perhaps through the stimulation of blood flow to the brain, according to some sources – but overindulgence increases the risk of cognitive impairment and dementia.

STAY IN TOUCH: See 'Loneliness and the network' on pages 85–91.

STOP SMOKING: Now. Today. Use the restrictions on smoking in public places as a reason, or the fact you don't want to smell like an ashtray. Or just stop because you want to reduce your risk of dementia, and the many other diseases you can opt out of by throwing away your cigarettes.

What is risk? If you cross a road just once a year, then you have a very low risk of being hit by a bus – but it could still happen. You can put all the above research findings together

– by going for a daily run with an optimistic and chatty friend before fortifying yourself on a diet rich in salmon, bananas and blueberries, washed down by a strong coffee and topped off with a glass of red wine – but that is not a guarantee of a dementia-free life. All the evidence suggests that these could be wise precautions that will lower your risk of developing dementia, but other factors are involved ... and we are learning more through the continuing but underfunded research into the causes of dementia.

the stages of dementia

'At the very beginning I didn't believe that you could possibly move all the way through these stages. But you do. Nothing is more certain than that.'

Sadly, dementia is a relentless decline, and it affects different people in different ways, some deteriorating faster than others. Health professionals divide the march of the disease into stages, but these are artificial classifications of symptoms, not real predictions of what will happen at a certain time. Giving a timescale for each stage can be misleading, as different types of dementia advance in different ways, and the boundary between one stage and the next is not clear-cut. The actual timeline will be continuous and often confused, and not everybody will show every symptom. People's response to dementia varies according to their emotional resilience and their physical robustness, and the progress of the disease will also depend on how much support and stimulation the person with dementia receives.

Most forms of dementia can be simply split into three stages: mild, moderate and severe (or early, middle and late). These labels can be useful as quick descriptions of how far the dementia has progressed, but a more involved breakdown of the symptoms of deterioration can be helpful in preparing for the future.

The most common dementia type – Alzheimer's disease – has been analysed and broken down into seven stages, according to the gradual loss of cognitive functions (this scale is known as the Reisberg Scale, or more grandly as the Global Deterioration Scale).

Stage 1 is the pre-dementia stage, where the thinking processes and memory work normally. Stage 2 includes some age-related lapses, such as forgetting names or where the car keys are, which are neither noticeable to others nor of real concern. By Stage 3 this has progressed to what is described as mild cognitive decline. Forgetfulness becomes more of a problem, the inability to concentrate or to find the right words may start to be apparent to others, and failures in planning or organisation may be evident. This stage is the first phase where clinical testing or a detailed medical examination might detect early evidence of Alzheimer's in some people.

'It's quite hard to get it into your head that you can't ask her questions about what's happened in the last five minutes or five hours. So much of life is built on that. "How are you?" "What did you do this morning?"'

In Stage 4, also known as the mild or early stage of Alzheimer's, the decline becomes more visible to others, to the extent that it can easily be detected in a simple test of cognitive performance. Memories of recent events become fuzzy, and intricate tasks become harder to complete. As awareness of the problem grows, people with dementia may start to retreat from friends and family, often denying any degeneration in their abilities, and the family may in turn find that friends and acquaintances drift away as social interaction becomes more awkward.

'The biggest shock to me was when they asked my wife what year it was, and she didn't have a clue. And it was a question that I would never have thought to ask her – and all of a sudden, the problem was clear. I didn't realise how far things had gone ...'

The cognitive functions decay further in Stage 5, or the mid-stage of Alzheimer's. There will be more troubling gaps in memory. Names and everyday details (such as home address or the date) will become elusive, and people may be stuck in a loop of repeating themselves over and over, evidence that their short-term memory is failing them. They are also likely to experience growing confusion, and there may be a need for support to help them manage simple daily activities, such as washing and dressing, eating or using the toilet.

Stage 6 represents the second part of the Alzheimer's mid-stage, and this may be when serious personality changes emerge. People may develop compulsive behaviours or even delusions, and they are highly likely to show signs of serious agitation and disruption to patterns of sleep. This is the stage where incontinence – either urinary, faecal or both – often becomes a persistent problem, and assistance with most of the simple activities of daily life will be required. This may include help with eating, as the ability to control cutlery deteriorates: cutting up the food so that it can be eaten with the fingers will help, or try mashing or using a food processor to make it easier to handle. People are liable to retreat further into their own bemused world as understanding and speech become increasingly difficult.

'As my wife's Alzheimer's developed, she started having small fits, going very stiff and slightly frothing at the mouth. It took me some time to realise what was going on – I thought she might be having a minor stroke – but the consultant said it's quite common. She was very distressed and it was quite a frightening experience. It totally exhausted her, and she had to lie down and sleep for a few hours afterwards to recover.'

Stage 7 – or late Alzheimer's – is a time of gradual shutdown and withdrawal. Interaction with the environment around the person with dementia fades in this final stage, and their ability to be understood and to control their own movements will slowly slip away. Almost totally dependent by now, many people lose weight dramatically and sink into apparent inertia, although restlessness and occasional bursts of aggression are not uncommon.

The other forms of dementia develop in different ways. Vascular dementia is often characterised by sudden steep declines, following repeated mini-strokes, although some people do lose abilities more gradually. The strokes may affect local areas of the brain, while leaving other parts functioning more or less normally.

In their later stages, dementia with Lewy bodies and fronto-temporal dementia develop in a similar way to Alzheimer's, but the earlier stages are different. Dementia with Lewy bodies shares symptoms with Parkinson's disease, and people with this form of dementia are prone to falls and often experience hallucinations. Fronto-temporal dementia is more likely to produce sharp changes in behaviour, with people often losing inhibitions and appearing selfish and rude.

CHAPTER 3

diagnosis and first steps

where to begin

If you have no experience of how dementia can change lives, take a moment to consider how much upheaval it can cause on both practical and emotional levels. At the core of dementia is a gradual retreat from the reality of now, and people with dementia will lose the capacity to make reliable and rational decisions based on all the facts. For trivial everyday matters, this simply means that the carers will need to guide the choices that need to be made. For the major issues – financial, health-related and legal affairs – the situation is more complicated, and formal safeguards exist to ensure that decisions are taken in the best interest of the person with dementia.

There are key elements to get in place in order to cope with what is ahead, and you will need to take action quickly. Documents will need to be signed and agreements made while the person with dementia can still make rational decisions – and while he or she can still demonstrate the mental capacity to do so. These are vital steps. Without a legal agreement authorising a carer to take decisions on behalf of the person with dementia, your freedom to act will be restricted by safeguards designed to protect those who cannot manage their own affairs.

Beyond the legal and administrative measures, it is important to look at the future as calmly as you can. Planning ahead is something everyone should be doing, and when the future involves dealing with the effects of dementia, that means planning the care that the person with dementia will need. Who is best placed to offer that care? And how can others help?

The big decisions fall into three areas: legal decisions, financial decisions and decisions on future medical care. But the first step is the diagnosis of dementia, and that will start with your local GP.

role of the GP

The hunt is on for a simple, reliable and inexpensive method of pinpointing the earliest signs of dementia. Medical researchers around the world are poring over clouds of data relating to the tiniest changes within the body, attempting to find a reliable and accessible 'marker', a detectable something that will give the earliest clear warning that the 'butterflies of the soul' – scientist and Nobel prize-winner Santiago Cajal's glowing description of the neurons in the brain – are under attack.

Until that becomes a reality, testing for dementia relies on spotting external symptoms – and they may start to emerge years or even decades after the hidden changes within the brain have begun. The first step in establishing whether a person's changing behaviour or memory lapses are simply normal age-related changes or signs of something more disturbing is a trip to the local surgery. With doctors under intense time pressure, it is not difficult to understand their unease about diagnosing something as veiled and undefined as the early stages of dementia, especially when the patient may be eager to conceal the symptoms.

Although heightened awareness of the growing numbers of people with dementia is improving detection, recent studies suggest that only about 46 per cent of people with dementia across the UK have been formally diagnosed – diagnosis rates are significantly higher in Scotland (64 per cent) and Northern Ireland (63 per cent). And a research paper published in 2007 suggests that the proportion of dementia patients receiving medication in the UK is less than half the level seen in other European countries.

Sandra, a busy GP who specialises in dementia cases, feels that the failure of some doctors to grasp the nettle of dementia may be due to their misgivings about how useful it is to determine the cause of cognitive decline and give it a name when there is still no cure. She believes that GPs are not unwilling to help, but they may be a little cynical about how much they can do to help, and they already have a lot of demands on their limited time.

'A lot of doctors were brought up to look at things purely from a medical model; and they sidestep

things that are a bit woollier and harder to diagnose precisely. I don't think doctors are very good at dealing with things they can't fix – and you can't fix dementia. Aricept is really just papering over the cracks. It may set things back a year, but it's not a cure.'

Most of the patients in Sandra's practice who bring up a concern about cognitive decline are unnerved by persistent errors or omissions at home or at work and are seeking either reassurance or help. They may know there is a problem – way beyond going upstairs and forgetting what they went up to do – but the root of the problem may not be dementia. The daily failings and frustrations that are haunting them and that are probably beginning to worry family and friends – the memory failures and the confusion – may simply be normal age-related decline, but they may also be signs of something other than dementia that needs medical attention. GPs will have to investigate whether the dementia-like symptoms perhaps stem from a bad reaction to some medication or are the result of an infection or stress. A variety of other diseases can mimic the feared effects of dementia: a deterioration in kidney function can interfere with abstract reasoning and reduce verbal memory performance, and diabetes can give rise to similar problems through damage to blood vessels in the brain and exaggerated swings in blood sugar levels. Even something as common as depression can give rise to worries about dementia.

'I get people coming to see me who think they've got dementia, but I only have to talk to them for five minutes to see this is depression. In depression, your concentration is poor, your decision-making skills are poor – and through fear they equate that with dementia. It's not that uncommon.'

Many carers will find that the doctor's first diagnosis is depression, as the patient withdraws from a world that is increasingly confusing and unsettling.

'About five years ago, we noticed that Dad started to get very down, didn't want to go and do things. We eventually got him to a doctor, and he diagnosed depression. I realise now that it's probably when it all started.'

Depression can, of course, coexist with dementia, and where the dementia is only suspected the doctor's strategy will often be to treat the depression first to allow further evaluation of the problem once the depression has been tackled.

Patients who are concerned about their failing mental powers and who are fearful of revealing the full extent of their problem will often delay mentioning their concerns about memory failings until the end of a consultation about another health issue. This leaves the doctor with very little time to assess whether there is a serious underlying problem, and the temptation might be to say, 'Oh, we all get like that as we get older.'

'If it crops up in the eighth minute [of a 10-minute appointment], I will usually say, "This is really important and I'd like to check it out properly," and ask them to come back. Of course, the difficulty with people who have memory problems is how to get them to come back for a review within, say, six months.'

Although GPs are becoming far more conscious of the importance of diagnosing dementia in its earliest stages, they still struggle to distinguish dementia from other problems, based on a rushed clinical assessment. A recent study by UK researchers suggests that GPs are now twice as likely to diagnose dementia where there is none, particularly in patients with depression or hearing problems, than to miss genuine cases of dementia. Deciding whether a poor cognitive performance amounts to dementia is much more complex when the patient is still perfectly capable of performing a simple daily routine, is a rare visitor to the surgery and lives alone. Only around one in three patients seeking help or reassurance related to dementia fears is accompanied to the appointment by a relative or friend, and that means in most consultations there is nobody present who can give independent insights into how well the patient is coping outside the surgery.

Most (though not all) of the people interviewed for this project felt their GPs had not been able to help significantly. So it's no surprise that a study of London GPs has found that fewer than one in three felt confident about their ability to diagnose dementia.

'Dad was getting more and more confused. He was taken to the doctor a few times and was told it was nothing to worry about – it's just what happens as you get older. He did have a way of being incredibly switched on when in front of the doctor, with no issues at all about whatever he was asked. So by the time he was diagnosed he was quite far gone.'

All GPs can really do is assess how confused a patient appears to them by briefly checking their powers of attention and concentration through tests of their information-processing and thinking skills. Several standard tests available to GPs, but the one most commonly used is the mini mental state examination (MMSE). This consists of a few relatively straightforward tasks and questions designed to evaluate uncomplicated mental processes, including testing short-term memory and general awareness of current events.

The official guidelines for doctors emphasise that this brief cognitive testing should be used merely in deciding which patients should have a more searching assessment, rather than as a full and final diagnosis in itself.

Sandra acknowledges the shortcomings of the testing, but still feels it has a useful function.

'These MMSE tests are limited in lots of ways, but they're very quick to do, and you just get an idea of how the patient is functioning. Is there definitely a problem here? Or is there no problem?

Or might there be a problem? That's as useful as they often are really.'

A few people take on the challenge of these tests and can rise to the occasion, summoning all their charm and persuasiveness to mask their confusion.

'She was a very forceful personality, and presented very well. Right to the end, she had extraordinary moments of lucidity. She could hold a perfectly normal conversation with you for half an hour, and you would wonder what everybody was fussing about.'

Others appear to be more intimidated. Think back to your schooldays when the people who relished the exams were usually the ones who were confident that they knew the answers. For the rest, exams were sometimes hard brushes with reality that risked exposing their ignorance. Now just imagine how intensely grim it must feel to be put through a test of your brain functions where giving the wrong answers will push you down into the 'dementia class'. It's no wonder that most people will find the process of being tested intensely stressful and confusing.

The MMSE assessment is scored out of 30, and – just like in school – high scores are good. The patients whom Sandra sees, who are concerned about their memory letting them down, are probably scoring about 25 or 26 out of 30.

'That's the level of everyday forgetting that we all do, and they just need reassurance that it's not more serious than that. It's only when someone is scoring 22 or 23 that we think of referring them for more testing.'

If GPs suspect their patients are showing symptoms of either mild cognitive impairment (poor memory functions, but not bad enough to interfere with everyday tasks or with reasoning skills) or dementia, they will probably be referred to a specialist assessment service for further study. Patients who are not referred for further assessment may find that the GP will ask to see them again in a few months so that their progress can be monitored.

GPs are encouraged to share the diagnosis of dementia with carers and family, but it can be done only with the permission of the patient, and that is sometimes not easy to obtain. Whether through embarrassment at the stigma of mental decline or fear of what may lie ahead, elderly patients often feel that their condition is a predicament that they wish to face alone.

The confidentiality that is part of the doctor–patient relationship becomes a barrier to establishing the facts, according to many carers, especially where there is denial of the problem. The patient's unwillingness or inability to share the doctor's views or advice with his or her carer and family can make visits to the surgery frustrating for those who are trying to understand how serious the situation is and how they can best give support.

Michael's mother would insist on going to see the GP or consultant by herself, and after each visit she refused to share with her family anything that had been said by the doctors.

> 'So there was Mum, whose brain was fragmenting badly, coming out of the surgery unable to remember anything that had been said – or she'd have a different spin on it. And the doctor wouldn't talk to my father at all. The whole issue of confidentiality is critical. You just need to be able to talk to the doctor and find out what's going on. Doctors should at least be able to talk to the carers in the family or someone whom they know has the interest of the patient at heart. She may be all right for the few minutes he sees her once a month, but a lot of the time she plainly isn't.'

And even when the person with dementia does allow a friend or relative to sit in on a consultation, that person is sometimes reluctant to ask the probing questions that need to be answered, which makes the task of finding where to go for help and what services are available in each area extremely difficult.

> 'My father couldn't ask because he couldn't talk to the doctor without my mother there, and she wouldn't have wanted him to ask. But even the people within the system appear to be ignorant of what help is on offer. And I really don't think that their doctor would actually have known much about what help was available.'

Some doctors will feel the need to push gently beyond the guidelines where it is clear that informally sharing their advice and recommendations with family carers would lead to better care for their patient. Some GPs even offer to tell the patient's carer first, so that he or she can break the news to the person with dementia.

When James went to the surgery with his mother for her assessment, the doctor asked if she'd like to hear the diagnosis or wait outside while she spoke to her son. Knowing how it would crush her to hear how far the degeneration had progressed, James had hoped she would let him face the verdict on his own, but she chose to come in and hear it herself.

'I think it was a shame, but of course it's her right to choose, and she made the decision in that moment, which I had to accept. But the diagnosis hit her really, really hard. We had lots and lots of tears for ages afterwards, terrible problems with confusion, and her saying she did not want to live.'

Hearing the results of the testing can be traumatic, whether the diagnosis was expected or a complete shock, and all the carer's diplomatic skills may be called upon to deal with the consequences.

Gerry found himself having to reassure his father that the diagnosis of dementia was the beginning of the fightback, not the end of hope.

'After the diagnosis, Dad was fuming. I asked whether anything had really changed, and he said,

"Absolutely! I've got dementia now!" So I asked if it made any difference. "Do I treat you any differently? You're the same person, but somebody has stuck on a label to help us deal with this problem"'

Kate was upset by the limited help that they got from the GP when her mother was diagnosed with dementia, but she accepts that he probably felt he was doing all he could. She feels that he was working within a system that fails to address the needs of people with dementia, where the whole family is involved in the care and the coping.

'In some ways I'm being critical of him, but it's the system not the individual. I know from our discussions that he was definitely not following the rules on confidentiality, and he went way beyond the call of duty in helping my father cope. I know he's a good man, but the system doesn't lend itself to clear and simple lines of communication or accountability.'

What Kate found most frustrating in her dealings with the authorities was the confusion and fragmentation – different bodies offering different services with no communication or coordination between them. At no point in her journey through dementia did she feel that there were clear signposts to help them find their way, and she argues that the GP's surgery should be the source of accurate information.

'If each GP practice had a booklet that explained what you can do if you or one of your relations have dementia – these are the options, these are the courses of action, these are the nursing homes, this is how you can contact the carers, this is who to go to for help with funding – that would be really, really helpful.'

denial

Medical intervention to deal with dementia is often most effective when it is provided early in the development of the disease. Yet the person who is almost always the first to sense the earliest hints of dementia – and that is the person trying to remember who you are, what day it is or where he or she lives – is sometimes the least inclined to seek help, and will disguise the symptoms and deny the diagnosis.

To understand this denial, imagine how things look from their viewpoint. Dementia is a fatal disease, and it will lead inexorably to the opposite of the tidy death most people would wish for – which is a calm end, without being a burden to anyone. Denial of a dementia diagnosis is a fightback, a refusal to lie down and just give in, and a last-ditch hope that it could be something else.

So how should you react when your loved one denies that anything is wrong? Well, the traditional Freudian belief is that denial must be confronted and conquered. The more modern view is less harsh, seeing denial as a coping mechanism. It's not regarded as a barrier that has to be broken down, but simply as evidence that the patient is not equipped to deal with the situation. When we cannot face what is put before us, denial is the easiest option and the only refuge.

It's not only the person with dementia who finds sanctuary in denial. Only years after his father died did Mark realise that he had probably been suffering from dementia, and that Mark's mother had refused to accept it and had tried to hide it. Curious comments that his father used to make were just glossed over, or perhaps they were subtle jokes. When his father suddenly asked him one Sunday if he'd enjoyed the local football game yesterday, was that a dig at Mark's infrequent visits home, or evidence that his brain was dancing between now and decades earlier? The truth that Mark discovered was that his mother had felt that her husband's strange behaviour was 'shameful', and so she had done everything she could to avoid the two of them being tarred with the stigma of mental illness, shielding him from scrutiny and difficult questions as he retreated into his inner world.

When his wife's dementia advanced to the stage of needing full-time professional care in a care home, Alan knew that the husband of a woman a few doors away had recently been diagnosed with dementia and started on medication, so he offered his help and support.

'I asked her if she wanted to have some of my books explaining dementia and how to care, but she just clenched her teeth and said, "I don't want to know anything about it. I don't want to know

what is going to happen, I'm just going to let it happen." Well, it's her choice ... but I walked away shaking my head, because I think the more you know about it, the better prepared you are.'

Why not try to look behind the denial at the fear that unleashes this defence mechanism to shut out a prospect that is too appalling to deal with? Denial is a self-protective reflex, ruled by the instinctive view that blanking out the threat is the only chance of survival, so a direct attack may only ring more alarm bells and spark a more aggressive defence. From the outside, denial can look as silly as the ostrich's mythical 'head-in-the-sand' reflex, but from the inside, that denial may be simply the last line of defence against just giving up. Do you really want to take that away?

Liz remembers her father's forceful personality and his refusal to acknowledge that he wasn't on the ball, even when the family tried to tell him he was suffering from dementia.

'He could be very assertive, and would deny any problem whatsoever. So the doctor was looking to treat him for depression, because he told him he was depressed because of a bad marriage! That was his spin, his way of dealing with it: he absolutely knew his brain was going, but he would deny it and say it was his wife's fault.'

From the first signs that his mother's awareness of the world around her was becoming foggier, Chris always worried about what was going on inside her head. But she rebuffed his attempts to help, and his father just wouldn't confront her.

> **'Both of them kept up the pretence that everything was fine. And I don't know to this day whether my mum really knew that was what she was doing. Perhaps she had decided that if everyone thought life was normal, then she could hold us all at bay until the end – which is what happened. My dad was complicit in not allowing us to challenge her. He was protecting her, and giving her what I think he felt was her dignity.'**

Part of the frustration of denial for the family and friends of the 'denier' is that they feel excluded at a time when they are desperate to be 'allowed in' to help. Unable to discuss and share the issues, they cannot know what is going on inside the head of their loved one.

> **'She did once tell a cousin who was very close to her that her brain was fuzzy and she didn't know what was happening to her. And she woke up occasionally in the night, sobbing, not knowing where she was or who she was, saying "This is awful ..." But then it was all put away, and not dealt with.'**

One best-practice approach in psychotherapy is to view someone's denial as a vital protective mechanism, much as an electrician might regard a fuse. If a fuse blows, then the circuit is shut down as a measure of self-protection, because the load being placed on that element is just too overpowering and would damage the whole system. Denial can persist until people are ready and able to face their truth; but when that truth is their own cognitive decline, some people may never reach that stage.

Is there a subtler approach that could come in 'under the radar'? Maybe what's needed is a hug (metaphorical or actual) rather than a full-frontal assault. It's terrifying to know that you're losing control of everything you do or think, and to accept that fate passively would be like giving up, acknowledging that all is lost and that the end credits are set to roll. Challenging the denial might squash the fragile hope that keeps total despair at bay. Yes, it might be easier for the carer if the person with dementia accepted the diagnosis ... but nobody said this would be easy; and the acceptance would probably be forgotten within minutes.

Instead of demanding acceptance of the diagnosis, Carolyn suggests embracing the denial.

> 'I can see no point in making Mum unhappy by getting into a row and saying, "Yes, you have got dementia," over and over again. So I just say, "You get confused. It's because you're getting older," and that's what she wants to hear. She still denies having dementia, so we agree that she just "gets confused", and she's happy with that.'

And nobody will deny that 'happy' is good. Or will they? There are at least two conflicting views on the benefits and dangers of denial in dementia. A genuinely sensitive and caring doctor gave this opinion on how to deal with people who come to the surgery troubled by fears that their memories are becoming increasingly unreliable.

> 'There's such a stigma and fear of dementia that people often won't use the word. So I use it early on, because when someone comes in worrying about their memory, they are worried – or perhaps a relative is worried – that they have got dementia. So if you don't use the word "dementia", you're just playing games. A lot of people seem to believe that if you don't mention something that people are anxious about, they will stop being anxious about it.'

Contrast the pained view of an equally sensitive and caring husband, who had to take his wife to the surgery and deal with her rigidly frightened and stony-faced reaction to being repeatedly told her fate.

> 'The professionals all say you should tell people. But everybody I've talked to agrees that they haven't got a clue! It takes days for her to get over going to these damned professionals because it upsets her. She basically doesn't want to hear that she's got dementia. It's like a death sentence.'

Who should get the last word on the merits of denial, the professionals or the carers? Perhaps a carer who was given heartfelt and very direct advice by a specialist geriatrician can bridge the gap. When Elizabeth expressed her concern about her parents trying to carry on as normal instead of facing up to a stark reality, she was countered with what she described as a 'very powerful comment'.

> 'Back off! They are your parents and this is their issue, not yours – so don't interfere. They are grown-up people, and if your mother chooses to be in denial, and your father chooses to go along with her on that, then it is their business, not yours ...'

legal

> 'Power of Attorney is the single most important thing – I can't emphasise it enough, especially if the husband has dementia, because the bank account is often in his name. And you cannot gain access to that bank if the person is no longer able to sign, so how does the wife get money? It just becomes an impossible situation ...'

When you suspect that a loved one might be suffering from dementia, one of the most important measures to put in place is the legal framework that will allow somebody else to take important decisions when that person loses the mental capacity to manage his or her own affairs.

The power that is granted is called a Lasting Power of Attorney, and there are two types: one for decisions relating to health and welfare (how and where medical care should take place, which medical interventions should be made or not made), and one for property and financial affairs (paying bills and taking money-related decisions). There are safeguards throughout the process to protect the interests of the donor (the person giving the power to act on his or her behalf): at least one independent person must certify that the donor understands the nature of the document and that no fraud or pressure has been used to persuade the donor to sign; the donor can list people who must be informed and invited to voice any concerns before the power is exercised; and the documents have to be reviewed by the Office of the Public Guardian before the power to act is granted.

The earlier you can do this, and the more you can make it feel like a natural age-related precaution, the easier you will find it. You may find that the dementia makes your loved one suspicious and possibly unwilling to get tied up in legal processes that he or she cannot fully understand. As the illness clouds comprehension, the person with dementia may seek to avoid any new and complex issues, fearing that a diminishing grasp on what is happening will be exposed. You may need to use subtle encouragement to overcome this reluctance, perhaps by showing your own willingness to go through what you regard as a natural process.

William, who was caring for his wife, told her that they should both tidy up their legal affairs as they were getting older.

'I said anything could happen to either of us, so we should make sure that our wills are up to date and we should give Power of Attorney to each other too. Then when we went to see a solicitor, I told him quietly that Power of Attorney for my wife should go to me and then to our children, but my Power of Attorney should go directly to the children.'

These coaxing subterfuges will, of course, be easier in some relationships than in others, and more successful at certain stages of the disease's development. The key point is that you should take these steps as soon as you can. However painful and unpleasant it is today, it will be worse next week. And if you do not manage to take out Power of Attorney while the person with dementia is still legally capable of agreeing to it, then you may find yourself stuck in the slow and expensive process of having to apply to the Court of Protection for the authority to manage his or her financial matters.

When she agreed to give her children Power of Attorney over her affairs, Barbara's mother found the whole experience very upsetting and felt it undermined her sense of herself and her abilities.

'But she's so glad now that we made her do it, because she has no worries about paperwork and she trusts me and my brother to make the right decision for her. Once she had actually got past that point of handing over the responsibility to us two, she felt absolutely fine.'

You can download the form to complete, and comprehensive guidance notes on how to do it, from the internet (go to www.gov.uk/power-of-attorney/overview). Read through the form and the guidance notes very carefully so that you understand what you are undertaking, and be sure to think through the consequences. The agreement that you are making is, of course, a binding legal document, and it must be completed with care. You may decide that a good friend is all you need to help you answer the questions and fill it in properly. But remember that if the form is wrongly completed, then it could be rejected at the point of registration – and that will mean starting all over again. If in doubt, find someone qualified to look it over and give you reassurance – that may mean asking someone at a Citizens Advice Bureau, or contacting a solicitor.

financial

'Help is on its way...' You're not expecting the cavalry, but help is on offer in the form of benefits that are paid out to help people living with dementia.

Attendance Allowance is the oddly named benefit payable to people aged over 65 who are living with a substantial disability and need some long-term help with their personal care (such as washing, dressing, eating or using the toilet) or require supervision (for their own safety or for other people's safety, including where it's related to taking medicine). You will need to fill in a form detailing what daily help the person with dementia requires and to supply contact details for their GP or other medical personnel.

There are two levels of payment: the lower rate is for people who need help during the day or at night, and the higher rate is for those who need both daytime and night-time care. The payments are tax-free and are neither means-tested nor dependent on having paid a certain amount of National Insurance contributions. Unless the person is in the final months of a terminal illness, the allowance is only paid after help has been needed for six months, but you can apply at any time before that point if you believe that the need for help will continue past the six-month period, as is likely in cases of dementia.

The Department for Work and Pensions claims that applications will be processed within 40 working days, and payments will be backdated to the date when you make the claim (that's either from when they receive your form or from when you call the helpline), subject to the six-month qualification noted above. A successful claim for Attendance Allowance will unlock your access to other financial help, such as Carer's Allowance (see page 72) and a reduction in Council Tax bills (see page 74), so it is important to get your claim in as early as possible.

There are several ways of getting hold of the application form. With a computer you can either download it and print it out, or complete the form online (go to www.gov.uk/attendance-allowance – read through the notes and see the page on how to claim). A computer-free alternative is to phone the Benefit Enquiry Line on 0800 882200 (that's the number for England, Wales and Scotland; in Northern Ireland the number is 0800 220674 – and textphone numbers are also available) and ask them to send you a form and information about it in the post. As long as you complete and return the form within six weeks, your application will be dated from when you made the call.

Nobody likes filling in complicated forms, but sometimes forms need to be lengthy because we live complicated lives. The application for Attendance Allowance consists of 15 pages of notes and 28 pages for you to fill in but, in a world that's short of good news, rejoice that it's three pages shorter than it used to be (although the current edition claims the form has only 27 pages) and the language is pretty straightforward. The pages of notes list the documents and information you will need to have at hand to complete the form – such as contact details for the GP and the name of any medication the person you are caring for may be taking. You may wish to ask a friend to help you if official forms give you a headache. You can also get some help on the phone if you are not confident about filling in the form yourself – the Benefit Enquiry Line will guide you through completing the form to ensure you get everything in the right place.

If the person with dementia is under 65, then the relevant benefit is a new entity called a *Personal Independence Payment*, details of which are available from the Disability Benefits Helpline on 08457 123456.

If you're spending more than 35 hours a week caring for someone with dementia who is in receipt of Attendance Allowance, then you may be eligible for *Carer's Allowance*. You don't have to be living with the person you're caring for, and you don't have to be related. However, you do have to be over 16 to apply, and you may not be eligible if you're in full-time education or earn more than £100 a week. Also if you're already receiving certain other benefits – including a state pension or incapacity benefit – which are equal to or more than the current rate of Carer's Allowance, then you may not get this payment. The calculations are pretty intricate, so if you want to know how this allowance will work with other benefits, you'd be wise to ask for advice from an expert (and that might mean the Benefit Enquiry Line, see pages 71–72 for telephone numbers; or a Citizens Advice Bureau; or just a clever friend who is willing to find out for you) before you make the application.

As with Attendance Allowance, you can apply online (www.gov.uk/carers-allowance/how-to-claim) if you're at ease with doing that, but you will need your National Insurance number handy, and you may be asked to send documents, such as accounts or a marriage certificate, by post to support your claim. (If you prefer, you can take your personal documents to a Jobcentre Plus where they can be copied and sent on to the Carer's Allowance Unit.) If you're happier filling out a paper form, you can either download one (go to the website noted above, and download DS700, or DS700SP if you receive a state pension) and print it out, or you can call the Carer's Allowance Unit on 0845 608 4321 and ask them to send you a form.

If you are caring for one or more people for more than 20 hours a week, you may also find that you are entitled to *Carer's Credit*. This is a top-up credit to make sure there are no gaps in your National Insurance record while you are taking on caring responsibilities, so that your entitlement to a state pension is not affected. You'll need to be over 16 and under state-pension age, and the people you're looking after must get either the Personal Independence Payment or Attendance Allowance.

Once it has been established that the person with dementia is entitled to receive Attendance Allowance, it may also be possible to knock a hole in their *Council Tax* bill. A couple living together, with one caring for the other who has dementia and receives Attendance Allowance, will be eligible for a 25 per cent discount. If the person with dementia is living alone, then there should already be a 25 per cent discount, but the receipt of Attendance Allowance may entitle that person to a full exemption from the tax. You will need to contact your local authority for details, as the eligibility criteria tend to vary in different areas, and your local authority will help you make an application.

driving

'The next thing was that the local GP stopped him from driving, which was a big thorn in his side, because he lost a huge part of his independence. He complained that he'd been driving for so many years, and was taught to drive in the army, but he didn't realise that none of that mattered at all. We were on the slippery slope then …'

Passing the driving test is one of the defining moments of growing up, a milestone in young people's quest for independence. And just as being handed your driving licence can open up a new world for a teenager, having that freedom taken away can be a devastating blow, and can feel like a heartless nudge towards helplessness.

Christine's mother had always been a very careful driver, and she took the withdrawal of her licence very badly.

> **'It was something she was really, really proud of, especially all the driving she had done as a Wren in the war. She started saying, "If I can't drive, I might as well be dead"'**

The proportion of people aged over 70 who still hold a driving licence has risen from around 15 per cent in the 1970s to nearly 50 per cent in the first decade of this century. Experienced drivers often describe the process of driving as almost automatic, but it relies on a web of interconnected elements. Our senses must detect other road users and potential hazards, our brains in both conscious and unconscious modes must process mountains of incoming data and our bodies need to react in a highly trained and skilled manner.

With all those strands working together, we can successfully navigate our way through the dangers of everyday traffic; but when that network breaks down, driving becomes infinitely more hazardous.

Priya was growing quite alarmed by her husband's driving, to the point that she started to find ways of preventing him from using the car.

'He arrived home one day and said that something strange had happened on the way. "I was on the roundabout up there and I suddenly did not have the slightest idea where I was going ... and I was scared!" he told me.'

The organisation entrusted with deciding whether or not drivers with specified illnesses can be allowed to retain their licence is the Driver and Vehicle Licensing Agency (DVLA). They must be informed when a driver is diagnosed with dementia – failure to do so is a criminal offence – and you should also inform the insurance company. But a diagnosis of dementia does not mean an instant ban from driving, although licences to drive commercial vehicles will be revoked if there is a likelihood of impaired driving performance. If the person with dementia wishes to carry on driving a car or motorcycle – and some 10 per cent of people with dementia do still drive – then the DVLA will ask that person's GP or consultant to report on the patient's ability to drive safely, looking at his or her comprehension of risks and perceptual awareness. Having reviewed that report, the DVLA may require the person with dementia to take a driving assessment at an approved mobility centre before deciding whether to grant a short-term licence or to require the driver to send in his or her licence. If the DVLA's decision is to allow the person with dementia to carry on driving, then that will normally be subject to an annual medical review.

There's evidence to suggest that most people with dementia give up driving before they have an accident, perhaps because their horizons shrink and the desire to go out just dries up.

This was what happened to Trevor's mother, whose driving was starting to be a cause for concern.

> 'We had been getting a bit anxious about it and then one day she just stopped driving. A month or two passed, and then the car needed to have its road tax renewed, and we decided we should sell it – she wasn't happy about not having a car, but she agreed that she wasn't using it.'

Concerned relatives often question the ability of someone showing signs of dementia to drive responsibly and safely. Christine is convinced that her mother should have been stopped earlier because she had lost her ability to make decisions and often had no memory of where she was going, which made her a very unpredictable driver.

> 'She came to visit us in London, but she drove to a flat that we had left eight years earlier. She got completely lost and then drove home, but by then we had reported her as a missing person.'

Christine discussed her mother's driving with her GP, pointing out that she was on a cocktail of medicines for various ailments, but he seemed dismissive of her worries.

> 'He said, "Oh, she's only driving around the village." But if anything unexpected had happened on the road – somebody suddenly doing something

different, or roadworks with a diversion – goodness knows what would have happened.'

Many partners of people with dementia hope that a doctor will take on the tough task of advising their loved ones to hand over their car keys. Janet was disappointed that the specialist who saw her husband allowed him to carry on driving, because she had seen his uncertainty at the wheel when he suddenly had no idea where he was.

'It was a problem with what I call his spatial awareness. He'd be driving somewhere we knew quite well and he would just blank out, not knowing whether to turn left or right. So I was taking on as much of the driving as I possibly could without having a direct confrontation with him.'

Sometimes that uncertainty does cause the serious accident that carers fear, and the result can be enormously upsetting for everyone involved. When Kevin's father froze in the middle of turning right at a T-junction, his car was hit by another vehicle and ricocheted into a pedestrian, who was badly hurt. Witnesses agreed that the accident was his fault and he was at risk of being prosecuted for dangerous driving.

'I asked the police what would satisfy them and be within the law, and they finally agreed that if he gave up his licence they would let him off with a warning. As far as my father was concerned,

it was a pack of lies. Somebody was out to get him, there was nothing wrong with his driving and it was totally the other person's fault.'

Ian's wife was determined not to give up driving in spite of her dementia. Even a serious stroke, which robbed her of her confidence on the road, did not dent her determination to carry on. When Ian turned to their GP for advice, he was surprised at the doctor's response that driving made her happy, without apparently considering the risk to others.

'He did finally tell her she shouldn't drive any more, and she cried for ages – she didn't get out of bed for two days because she was so upset. In the end I told her the car was getting beyond repair, and she did accept it eventually.'

People with dementia can sometimes be persuaded to use a less dangerous way of getting around by carers emphasising the difficulty of parking or the slowness of traffic, or praising the bus service into town. But some carers find that a 'white lie' is the only way they can prevent someone who is no longer capable of driving safely from using the car. Subterfuges such as 'losing' the keys, or booking the car into a garage for repairs, are desperate and temporary solutions. If, however, you are convinced that someone with dementia is a danger on the road, and you have tried every other means of dissuading them from driving, then one GP advises calling the DVLA and voicing your concerns – anonymously, if you wish – so that they can be asked to take a driving assessment to determine objectively whether or not they are safe behind the wheel.

in their shoes

Caring for somebody who is being slowly consumed by dementia is both daunting and exhausting. Those feelings are intensified when that 'somebody' is a loved one – a parent, a partner, a sibling or a friend. It's an experience that will test your patience and your temper to breaking point, and there will be times when you just want to scream and run away. One way of avoiding this crisis is to harness family and friends to work together and share the responsibility. Carers have also found that seeing the world from the point of view of someone with dementia can work wonders – almost literally – in smoothing out difficulties. So ... put yourself in their shoes for a few moments, and imagine their thoughts and anxieties.

'It strips away the self. You have no control over it. It must be torture ...'

What goes on inside when the certainties of a lifetime disappear, when objects conspire against you and the simplest words fade away as you reach for them? And, worst of all, how does it feel when every moment is infected by the fear – and it's slowly becoming a certainty – that you're losing your mind? Road-test their fragmented reality for a few moments, as it swims in and out of coherence.

Normally, when you close your eyes and let your mind wander, you still have a hold on reality. If you open your eyes, you are once again secure in the 'here and now', back from wherever your thoughts carried you. But when the functioning of the brain is affected by dementia, there is no safe return from those mental wanderings, no signposts pointing back to a calmer sanity. Although it may feel like a nightmare, nobody is going to wake you from your anxious struggles and comfort you. As the neural networks within your brain fragment, your thoughts and perceptions can go astray, filling your consciousness with the oh-so-real ghosts of forgotten events and long-dead people. Doors will open onto jarring and unexpected realities, a lifetime away from where you thought you were. Familiar faces from your distant past will laugh at you and deny their identity, pretending to be sons or daughters that you don't have. Strangers, who may claim to be your spouse, will offer to perform intimate services, and will prevent you leaving to find your 'real home'. Your tensions, your panic, your fears will multiply, as everything and everyone will seem to be against you, doubting you, challenging you and imposing an alien reality on you.

And what of those people around you who you rely on to help you out of this hell? Why do they believe that pointing out your errors will restore you to coherence, and that correcting you will cure you? Can they not understand why you retreat from a world that is itself going crazy, repeatedly ambushing you with its channel-hopping delusions? Do they not expect you to fight against the 'Etch-a-Sketch' wiping of everything you know, everything that defines 'you'? Is this my house? And why do they keep asking me if I'd like a cup of tea? Do I like tea? Have I just had a cup? So many questions … but the apparently simple answers may be lost for ever in the tangles of your fogged cognition.

Now imagine the bravery and faith that you would need to hand over all responsibility for your cognition and information processing to A. N. Other, without losing all hope. Try it now. Accept unreservedly that someone else – perhaps someone half your age, perhaps your equally fallible spouse – is right and you are wrong about the most basic things. Yes, you put the car keys in the freezer. No, the person you were just talking to was not real. Yes, you did park the car at the supermarket and then report it stolen. No, you are not an intelligent being but someone who is drifting at the mercy of misfiring neurons …

Understanding is the key. If you can communicate a sense that you understand where the dementia has taken your loved one, then perhaps that person can feel that the burden is being shared. If your loved one can believe that your feelings towards them haven't changed, that there is still the same unequivocal love and support on offer, then perhaps he or she will agree that you can fight this most effectively together. So if something imagined or real is persistently nagging away at your dementia-affected charge, would it not be helpful for you to agree that 'something should be done', so that you can shoulder the responsibility to sort it out?

'What has helped me enormously is acknowledging that my mother is never going to come back into my world. So if we are ever going to meet – at least

emotionally – then I have got to go into her world. So when she looks around and frowns, making that face that means "This just isn't right", I join in. I say to her, "It's a bit of a muddle." And she says, "Yes, it's a bloody muddle," and we're all right.'

By working alongside her mother rather than asking what is making her frown, Angela is able to pick up on the subtle cues that may only be visible to someone who knows her mother well. And instead of trying to 'jolly her along' – which might put emotional distance between her and her mother, suggesting that she is 'in the wrong' – she instinctively sides with her, recognising and echoing the feelings that are troubling her.

'Little things like that have been a godsend, saying the thing that is going to calm her down and take away her anxiety and her terror … or simply agreeing with her, where to disagree would matter and where agreeing doesn't matter. So when she looks at some person across the room and says, "That's a horrible person," all of me wants to tell her not to be so judgemental, but what I say is, "Yes, I can see what you mean …" and just agree. And then it's all right. We can move on.'

Martha sighs as she thinks back to conversations she and her husband had when he was clearly struggling to keep track of events and people around him. Now that she has learnt more about what was probably going on in his brain during those months, her memories of their time together are tinged with regret, and she is bitterly conscious that she could have handled things differently.

> 'I was cross with him for not engaging, and sad that I was losing that closeness that we had always had. I was trapped between all that sadness and crossness and not sure how to handle it, and I can see now that what I wasn't doing was giving enough in that period when he could have used some comfort, some interaction.'

Sometimes the best comfort you can provide for your loved one is the feeling that you are with them, beside them on their journey.

CHAPTER 4

care and community

loneliness and the network

'Basically she sat there from seven in the morning until seven at night, watching the TV and having nobody to talk to. I can't help feeling that it contributed to her developing Alzheimer's.'

Humans are – by and large – social beings. In the normal course of our lives we interact with a huge number of other people in many different contexts – at work, at play or in the necessary transactions of modern living, such as shopping. Those dealings with others may be entertaining or frustrating in themselves, but researchers are finding a hidden value in the stimulation that these exchanges provide. A study of older people in the US suggests that simple social activities, such as going on day trips or spending time with relatives or friends, can play a role in reducing the risk of cognitive decline. More than 1,100 people with no sign of cognitive impairment were monitored over five years, and subjected to a range of memory tests and analysis of their perception and visuo-spatial abilities. The investigation found that the people with the lowest levels of social activity were four times more likely to develop cognitive impairment than those who were the most socially active.

It is not difficult to understand that if you feel less sure of yourself than you used to, and are consumed by the fear that your cognitive powers appear to be fading away, then you would naturally be less tempted to take part in social activities. But what makes this study particularly interesting is that the researchers deliberately chose a methodology designed to exclude the possibility that the decline was the forerunner of, or the cause of, withdrawal from the activities. Their conclusion is that the inactivity and isolation seem to be leading to or precipitating the decline in cognitive powers, rather than the other way around.

Even if poetry brings you out in a rash, you may have heard John Donne's famous maxim 'No man is an island', and if the island you picture is buffeted by storms and isolated, then no person should be allowed to feel like an island. Yet one in five of Britain's older people has contact with friends, family or neighbours less than once a week – and one in ten has that sort of company less than once a month. Of course, being alone is not the same as being lonely. Positive and resilient individuals can be alone without being lonely, while people with depression or low self-esteem can feel lonely in a crowd. But if a person's main 'company' is the television set – as half of the older people in one survey confessed – then that person is likely to be lacking the stimulation that he or she needs.

When Stella's mother was widowed, she seemed to lose all hope and go into a slow decline. She moped around the kitchen, lamenting that there was nobody to cook for, and would simply wait all day on her own, brooding and withering. Stella would often come back from work to find her sitting mournfully on the doorstep, like a lost child.

'As soon as my father died, she started wishing she was dead. She had nobody to talk to at home. Most of her friends had moved away, and she wasn't a very social person. If it had happened the other way round – if my father had been still alive and she had passed away – he would have gone and made friends and talked to people, but she was very shy.'

David's mother never suffered from shyness, and when he began to worry that she was becoming increasingly lonely, she dismissed the idea impatiently. She insisted that she was part of a group who would regularly play cards together, but David discovered that her set of friends had largely abandoned her, with one exception.

'She was going down to the pub with this friend who had stuck with her, and they used to play cards with whomever they met in the pub, because she was much happier in the company of strangers

> than she was in the company of people she knew. When you're with people you've known for years, they reminisce, and Mum was finding that harder and harder. With her "mates" in the pub there were no demands on her to remember. So she actually lost contact very quickly with her "real" old friends.'

The breakdown of social networks has been linked with greater depression and alcoholism. But a recent study of adults aged between 50 and 68 showed how being lonely can have a direct impact on people's health. The study found that the people with the highest scores on measures of loneliness were also likely to have the highest blood pressure. More surprising, even to specialists in the care of older people, was the finding that the measured differences in blood pressure between lonely and non-lonely subjects were at their highest in the oldest age groups tested – in other words, the older the person, the worse the effects of the loneliness on blood pressure.

What is the distinction between being alone and being lonely? It's nothing but your state of mind, and yet that difference can be damaging to your health. Being alone is not a health risk in itself, but being lonely – whether that's passively pining or actively yearning for companionship – really is bad for you. A four-year study of older adults with a mean age of over 80 showed that lonely people had twice the risk of developing Alzheimer's disease compared to others described as non-lonely, regardless of physical problems or vascular risk factors. Research carried out on 2,000 elderly people in

Amsterdam has confirmed that loneliness – rather than objective measures of social isolation – does increase people's risk of dementia.

Loneliness and isolation can be as dispiriting and health-challenging for carers as it is for people with dementia. When Victoria's 89-year-old husband developed dementia, simply making himself understood became a trial. His speech degenerated into a few recognisable words marooned in a jumble of sounds, and silence spread through the house.

> 'That has been the most difficult part of all this for me. I can cope with the physical side of caring for somebody, but not being able to communicate with someone you've been married to for over 60 years ... well, it's really hurtful. I can go to the shop or pass somebody in the street and they will have a chat with me, but I come home ... and we can't talk about it.'

Even disciplined scientific research seems to suggest that being lonely has the effect of chilling your soul. People asked to estimate the ambient temperature after recalling a time when they were socially excluded found the room colder than those who had been asked to remember an experience of being included – it's mirrored in our language when we use the terms 'cold shoulder' and 'warm welcome'. Other research volunteers, who had been playing a computer-simulated ball-catching game in which some participants were 'thrown' the ball more often than others, were offered a choice of warm or cold drinks afterwards. Those who had been included in the game more often tended to choose cold (refreshing) drinks, while the group who had been thrown the ball less often (and therefore felt more excluded) were significantly more likely to choose a warm (comforting) drink.

Loneliness has been described as chronic distress with no redeeming features, and it can have real physical and medical results that go far beyond anything felt in simulated research. Anything that can be done to provide the emotional nourishment of true and valuable connections may be a real lifesaver for people like Victoria, caring for her husband with dementia. She describes how when she and her husband bought their house some fifty years ago, the road was full of young families who would meet while walking the children to school each morning. But once the wives learnt to drive and the children grew up, everything changed. Even the spindly trees lining the gardens grew and thickened, isolating each private rectangle of lawn and stifling the neighbourly chats over the fence. Big events, such as a street party for the Queen's Jubilee, briefly broke those barriers, but Victoria hasn't seen many neighbours since. 'I expect they've got families ...,' she muses.

Perhaps it's time for a revolution of kindness to break down some of those barriers by ringing some old people's door bells – but without running away afterwards! Once you realise that a regular five-minute chat with someone lonely, or an offer to put their bins out each week, or taking an occasional plate of those biscuits your children like to make round, or – insert your own ideas here – could prolong and enrich that person's life, maybe warding off dementia for a while, then even the busiest personal schedule might find a few otherwise wasted minutes to spare. And isn't it good news that you don't have to dive into a storm-tossed sea or fight your way into a burning building to be a life-saving hero? You can just stretch out a friendly hand wherever you are.

friendships

When the sergeant-major addresses the weary platoon and calls for 'volunteers for a working party' to take one step forwards, there are always canny old campaigners who will quietly take one step back, as a precaution against getting involved. Yes, of course you've heard it before, but like many old jokes, there's more than a little truth in it.

The truth is that until the people you love are felled by a crisis, you will never really know which of their friends will rush to help them back on their feet. A well-filled address book can feel like a sturdy defence against anything the world can throw at them, but not everybody on their list will be in a position to support them just when they need it most. For some, that's a matter of timing, as they may be consumed by their own problems. For others, it may be a case of mistaken identity – although your loved one had them down as 'friends', perhaps they had your loved one filed under 'acquaintances'. And a large third group may be squeamish about 'mental illness' or just frightened by the whole thing, and unsure how to help or where to begin.

When her mother was diagnosed with dementia, Karen hoped that her old friends would rally round in support. So she found some of their rejections intensely painful.

> **'Her best friend, whom my mother used to drive somewhere every week, apparently couldn't cope with what was happening to her, and she simply abandoned her. And Mum knew that she had abandoned her, and she found that totally devastating.'**

Knowing that her mother's old friends were falling away through embarrassment reminded Sophie of stories her mum had told her of the days when she had looked after children she had described as having 'mental problems'. When she used to take the youngsters into their little town to shop or just to look around, she noticed that the majority of her friends and acquaintances would pretend not to see her and cross the road to avoid the embarrassment of having to talk to the children.

> **'Exactly the same thing started to happen with my mum when my dad took her out in town. He could see the people they knew crossing the street because they didn't want to talk to her – simply because she would repeat herself – or because they didn't know how to talk to her. It made him feel so awful.'**

Looking back, Sophie feels sure that she and her father should have handled their friends differently, and got them 'on their side' earlier on. If her father hadn't felt so protective and hadn't been so determined to shield his wife from situations where she might feel embarrassed, then she believes a larger group of their friends might have stayed loyal.

'I think he didn't tell people she'd got dementia until it was too late, and that was partly because he didn't want to face up to it. So there was this gap where I think they probably lost a lot of their friends because my father didn't get in touch with them, and didn't want to tell people what was happening.'

With hindsight, Sophie is convinced that her father should have told friends the truth about what they were going through, and should have explained that they would still love to see friends if they could cope with the unusual behaviour that came with her mother's dementia. Then the ones who were prepared to ignore the repetition of this and the forgetting of that could still have stayed in touch. As it was, her father's loyalty and the protective barricades he built around his wife actually made them more isolated. Nevertheless, their core friends would not let them suffer alone and were a source of great strength until the end.

'Their oldest friends from when they were young were fantastic. There were a few couples who

stood by them all the way, and they would have lunch all together every week. And their neighbours – who they had had a few tricky times with over the years – turned out to be marvellously supportive.'

is honesty the best policy?

Whoever you're caring for, you may find that honesty is not the simplest way to achieve the desired outcome. Although telling the truth is admirable and desirable in most situations, it can be cruel and unhelpful for someone with dementia.

It's easier to cope with total honesty when you're feeling good. Researchers who invited people to choose 'truth' or 'happiness' discovered that those in a positive mood were more willing to accept the truth, whereas stressed or anxious people were more likely to seek happiness. It seems logical – if the familiar world around you has become unpredictable and confusing, ambushing you with a twisted reality, then it's a natural instinct to seek reassurance, stability and happiness before anything else. Now is not the time to be grappling with an enormous truth: that can wait until you're back in control.

When you share the true facts with someone, you are also sharing the burden of that truth and the responsibility of acting on it, and all that may be too much for someone with dementia to handle. To give calm reassurance that everything that can be done is being done may be more valuable and helpful than simply stating the facts to somebody who is in the grip of a disease that makes it impossible to process those facts in a rational way. Is that lying? No, says Eric.

> 'You don't really lie. You just use words to overcome a situation. It allows "the right thing" to happen without upset ... without upset for her, at least.'

But not sharing the truth goes against the natural flow of a relationship, and it can signal a decisive change of role. Whatever the nature of your relationship was – partner, child, sibling, friend – you are now 'the one who knows best' ... and that's a big, lonely responsibility.

Perhaps viewing it as a straight-forward choice between 'telling the truth' or 'telling a lie' is too simplistic, too black and white for a complex situation of shifting shades of grey. Choosing how to phrase the truth and selecting which portions of the truth to share are part of our everyday interactions with others. At work, at play and at home we moderate the truth with the best of intentions. For many carers, the experience of shielding someone from unpleasant and unhelpful truths is a throwback to the parent–child relationship; but now the roles are uncomfortably reversed, and it may be the turn of the child to protect an ailing parent from the cold fingers of reality.

Michelle has found herself using the same psychological approach with her mother that she used with her children.

> 'Sometimes, by just masking the bare truth, you can avoid unhappiness – and that's absolutely fine. It's simple diplomacy.'

You may find that you have to mask different levels of reality as the dementia progresses. Derek knew that his wife had always hated the thought of being put in a care home, but the time came when she needed more expert care then he could give her. When she moved into a care home nearby, she only felt calm when the whole family worked together to conceal the unpalatable truth from her. Although he hated misleading her, he knew it was the best solution for her.

> 'I used to go every night after work. I'd take her favourite things for us to eat, and when I put her to bed, I'd pretend that I lived there too. She'd ask, "Where are you going?" and I'd say I was going to my room next door, but she wouldn't see me in the morning, because I had to get to work early.'

Although most people tell the truth most of the time, almost all of us tell tiny white lies without malice to avoid someone else's discomfort. In the words of one psychologist, they 'grease the wheels', making life run more smoothly. To avoid causing unnecessary distress, Shirley felt she had to massage the truth of her mother's foggy memory of battling with paramedics and berating doctors in the local A&E department one night.

> 'She was angry in the morning, saying, "What was all that about? I told you never to take me to hospital!" So I said, "No, it was me. I hurt my arm and you came with me." My sister stared at me,

but I told her later, "This is what it is like. You have to go with what she thinks is real."'

When others become involved, masking the truth with good intentions becomes more problematic, and may go against professional ethics or policy. People concerned about an ageing relative's gradual deterioration often encounter reluctance to get a proper diagnosis, and may put pressure on the GP to invent a pretext for seeing the patient. This can put the doctor in an awkward situation, where the family's wishes may clash with the professional view of the best long-term outcome.

'With all these scary diagnoses like dementia, you end up with lots of "secrets and lies" going on – and it's very difficult when relatives say, "I don't want him to know, because he'll give up." They may be right, but I find they're usually wrong. You end up with nobody addressing the big issues, because then the patient might know that he or she has got dementia.'

Honesty and openness in facing up to a horrible reality may be the right choice in the earlier stages of dementia. There's a 'good honesty' in sharing your concerns with a loved one whom you feel is in trouble, in order to access better care and to release him or her from the loneliness of unshared fears. But later on, as the dementia clouds that person's reality, an unwavering focus on honesty can be cruel, as Ruth recalls from overhearing a conversation between her mother – who had dementia and was dying of cancer – and a specialist nurse.

'I remember my mother asking this nurse if she would get better and this nurse saying, "No, you won't ..." and my mother crying. Two minutes later she had forgotten what had been said, but remained fretful and anxious, knowing there was something awful in the air. Then she would repeat the question, and the nurse would say, "No, you're going to die quite soon," and she would cry again. These nurses have a policy of total honesty, but this repeated death knell was so insensitive. Whereas if she had simply said something like, "Well, we all die in the end, don't we?" it wouldn't have made her so sad and upset over and over again.'

Sometimes the traces of turmoil left behind by a disturbing real-life experience will resurface. Dementia may have eroded the true circumstances, but the feelings of fear or sadness often remain, like unexplained footprints in the snow. Betty's father committed suicide, and the shock of that episode was never far from the family consciousness. When her mother developed dementia, although she could no longer summon up the sad facts of what had happened, the inner grief and torment would emerge in periods of gloom and desolation.

'For three months she wasn't eating and for three months she was sobbing her heart out, saying,

"I want to die, I want to die. If I was braver, I'd kill myself." Then she'd look at me and ask, "Did somebody kill himself?" And I would say, "Yes," and she might or might not ask who, but I would never give her the information if she didn't ask me. These days she doesn't remember him, really. As her memory declined, she would ask how he died, but her doctor and I agreed that there was just no point in giving her details that are going to upset her even more ...'

who's in charge?

'As a carer, you have that tension between letting the person live their own life – and although it's not what you'd count as a normal life, they are actually quite happy, but you know there are risks attached – or choosing to take a more paternalistic approach, and saying they need a lot more guidance or supervision. The problem is deciding which is better. People get very agitated when someone gets a bit lost, but in a way Dad is quite happy. He's not really distressed by it at all.'

One of the difficult aspects of caring for someone with dementia is that there is no single set of rules, no textbook to lay down a trouble-free path that will work for everyone. All you can hope to find is a description of some of the obstacles you are likely to face and tips on how you might choose to avoid them. One of the knotty questions you will come up against in the early stages is how much you should intrude on the everyday existence of the person with dementia. How interventionist – or interfering – should you be? When should you think of taking the car away? How soon do you start to worry about the gas cooker being left on? And how will your worry affect the person with dementia?

> 'My brother and I had a long conversation with her today about how she really needs more help, and she looked quite puzzled. In her view she doesn't actually need any help at all. But all her neighbours are telling me of their concerns that in the afternoons she is at a loose end so she just wanders around and tries to have a chat with people.'

How do you balance a person's right to 'wander around' and 'chat with people' against your fears that they may endanger themselves and others? And should your view change because neighbours are suggesting that you're not taking proper care of them? Most people who care for someone living with dementia are more worried about their safety than about them being embarrassed. As Tom elegantly commented:

> 'I don't actually care very much if she walks around naked in the street one day – and there is a distinct possibility that she might do that – but I do worry that she's going to come to harm.'

A serious incident can of course change the rules completely, and what might have been seen as 'interfering' is transformed into a necessary precaution. Concern that her father's deteriorating memory was becoming a genuine danger was the trigger for Hazel's decision to move him out of the house he had lived in for decades.

'He nearly set his house on fire when he suddenly decided to light a fire in the grate, having forgotten that the chimney had been blocked up years earlier. I happened to phone him when the fire brigade was there. He told me they were there but he didn't know why they had come.'

Fear that someone with dementia will be more vulnerable to crime is one of the prime safety fears. Dementia can alter people's perception and judgement, and leave them open to exploitation by conmen, as Lillian discovered. Although her husband was usually a cautious person, he came back from the paper shop one day with a man whom she presumed had been a business acquaintance. She was surprised when her husband gave him a bundle of cash, but it was only after the man had left that Lillian realised he had been a stranger with a sob story, and that they had been conned.

'That was just so out of character for my husband. He would normally have been suspicious of anyone like that – and I suppose that was why I was taken in too.'

A recent study, in which subjects of varying age were asked to rate faces on a scale of trustworthiness, has confirmed that older people are simply more trusting of faces that quickly arouse suspicion in younger age groups. When brain activity was monitored while the faces were being judged, a distinct difference between old and young was noted. Part of the brain known as the anterior insula became active in the younger adults, particularly when a face was rated as untrustworthy, but little corresponding activation was seen in the older brains.

Citizens Advice agrees that people with dementia are particularly at risk from scams and fraud. One of their recommendations is that carers might help vulnerable people to sign up to telephone and mailing preference services that will help cut down on unsolicited telephone sales calls and unwanted 'special offers' in the post. Dealing with conmen who come to the door when the person with dementia is alone in the house is much trickier, as reminders about the dangers of being conned are not likely to be retained. Ensuring that cash, cheque books and credit cards are kept in a safe place might help avoid money being handed out, but if you believe that someone with dementia has been the victim of a scam or fraud, contact Action Fraud on 0300 123 2040. Action Fraud is the government agency responsible for fighting fraud and they promise an enhanced service to vulnerable people.

Jess became concerned that her mother was laying herself open to unscrupulous characters. Wishing not to be troubled by her house keys, which she kept mislaying, her mother would often go out and leave her front door open, claiming in justification that there were no burglars where she lived. Jess pleaded with her to take more care, and gave her a house key on a chain around her neck so that she would always have the key with her when she needed it.

> 'But now when she comes home and finds the door locked, she forgets she has the key around her neck and she goes and asks the builders working a couple of houses away to break into her house. They're nice strong men and she smiles at them, so they sometimes break into her house for her. And then I get anxious calls from some neighbours, saying they've found my mother and some men breaking into the house again.'

Taking steps to protect people with dementia from being robbed or worse is of course vital, but carers find a tension between being protective and being overprotective. Although it's a natural instinct when you find yourself slipping into this new position of responsibility to try to wrap your loved one in cotton wool, it is really important for his or her self-image and self-confidence to allow someone with dementia to preserve independence and stay motivated and active for as long as possible.

Dr Johnson once observed that nobody comments if a young person forgets something, but an aged person who does the same is mocked and seen as losing his memory. If we are looking for a fault, we usually find one. It leaps out at us, and treating it as evidence of a bigger problem can be a self-fulfilling prophecy. It's something that experts sometimes refer to as 'excess disability' – treating people as less capable than they really are has the effect of reducing their ability or willingness to act independently. Simply commenting or frowning when someone fails at a task, or avoiding giving them the task in the first place, can exacerbate a feeling of helplessness, according to Peter, who believes that giving his father an active part to play in the household actually makes him feel better.

'If he says, "Oh, let me do that," I let him now, rather than doing it myself, even though I know it's going to take twice as long for him to do it. It gives him a role, and that's important. I used to feel guilty about him doing the washing-up in the sink because we've got a dishwasher. But now I am happy to let him do it, because he feels he's contributing, and that is good for him. I think that's where they often get it wrong in some care homes, not understanding that, even though people are deteriorating mentally, they are still better off with something to do.'

Even though Tom's mother is moving into the advanced stages of dementia, she still has a fuzzy memory of the art and needlework that she used to enjoy, and keeping herself busy with that gives her great pleasure. So she will happily surround herself with her painting or needlecraft materials and sort them from one box to the other, and might then shuffle some of the bits into another box.

> 'She will just keep doing that for hours, all in a relatively contented way. Sometimes there's a bit of frustration there, because at the end of three hours, she might look at it and say, "This is such a mess. What am I going to do?" And she is quite capable of starting all over again unless you step in and distract her. So she can still occupy herself, with a vague notion that there's a purpose to it and she's going to paint something this afternoon – but she doesn't get that far any more.'

His mother's days tend to follow that pattern, a mix of different activities, with more beginnings than endings. When she's recounting what she has done, she will often fill in any lost hours with plausible activities that she might or might not have actually got round to.

> 'Every day I come home and she will tell me she's been out, taken the dogs out and had a lovely walk. It used to terrify me, because she really hasn't the capacity to control the dogs on leads any more, and I used to wonder if I should shut the dogs away – but thankfully it's all in her mind.'

titles and roles

> **'Your mother's reaction to dementia is to put her coat on, go outside and see who's there to talk to. And my mum's solution is to wrap herself up in bed and decide she's got a bit of gastric flu.'**

Offer somebody a glass of water, and that person might see the glass as half-empty. Others will regard it as half-full. And a third group may just wittily observe that the glass was too big or that you weren't very generous in filling it. If you look at any two individual people who are at the same broad stage of their dementia, then you are likely to find that they will respond to their gradual loss of abilities in totally contrasting ways.

> **'The two of them are so different in their attitudes. Your mother always says, "I keep forgetting everything, I get discombobulated ... but I remember my name and where I live." So she has an analysis of what is happening, but my mother tells us there is just nothing wrong.'**

The differences between those two mothers are probably just innate aspects of their characters that have always been there. Some forms of dementia, such as fronto-temporal dementia, can cause unexpected personality changes, dissolving the normal social restraints to produce strangely uninhibited behaviours. But however distorting or exaggerating the effects of dementia may be, the person inside is still very much the same. The person's character doesn't change.

'When she started losing her memory, Mum told me about a neighbour who was getting increasingly cranky, and she said something that I thought was very perceptive: "As people grow older, they don't really change. They just grow the same, only more so."'

Beth found her mother's comment a perfect description of how dementia had first affected her. She had never had a good sense of direction, and her dementia quickly accentuated that weakness, leaving her confused by new places, unable to find her bedroom or the kitchen on holidays, but still quite able to find her way around the familiar streets she had known for decades.

'Another thing she said was that when people grow old, some people end up anxious and depressed, and others become happy and forgetful – and we're lucky that she's one of the happy and forgetful ones.'

Attempts to cram people into our little mental pigeonholes usually land us in trouble, particularly if we prejudge infinitely variable human beings solely according to their age or their gender. The simplistic belief that if you like football you're a man and if you like cooking you're a woman was ridiculous long before Delia Smith showed you can like both; and there is enough variation within each gender or age category to make simple stereotypes woefully misleading. But consideration of the broadest, most generic characteristics of men and women in the age groups currently most likely to be living with dementia might throw light on the hidden feelings that may be haunting them, or the aspects of caring that they may find the hardest to manage.

So, using the crudest, most caricaturing brushstrokes, don't be surprised when men with dementia find it almost painful to ask for help. There is a male instinct that dictates that problems must be solved and should be solved, and failure to find that solution is just too shameful to contemplate. When men tackle run-of-the-mill tasks, failure is the foreplay to the ritual of 'blaming the tools'. But that's not an option in this case. When the tools that are letting you down are tools deep within yourself – your memory spluttering like an old lawnmower, your concentration dancing around you and then running off like an excited puppy – then the situation becomes dire. Nobody trains men to believe that it's acceptable to show when they're at their wits' end, or frightened or vulnerable. Some will share those feelings, but many will hide them away, and protect them with impatience and a growling introspection while the emotions fizz and bubble inside.

As carers, most men might feel able to keep the finances in order, whereas the gentler caring aspects of looking after a spouse and the house are possibly less familiar territory. Men may be less sensitive to slight nuances of behaviour, and helping a wife dress or do her make-up are not part of a man's core curriculum – but at least more husbands these days will be able to put a decent meal on the table. Unwilling to admit when they need help as carers, men can also be poor at gathering friends around for support – and, as friends, they are often more wary of 'interfering' by offering help to others.

And what of women? In couples facing the reality of dementia today, many of the women will have been in sole charge of the catering and cleaning, and they may find that relinquishing that role leaves them uneasy, but perhaps less explosively frustrated than men. Women are often more able to voice their emotional needs and this can allow them to express their concerns in a more open manner.

As women are often more familiar with a caring role, more at home with collaborative methods and more flexible in their approach to getting things done, women are likelier to establish a powerful network of supportive friends and deal more stoically with the stresses and exhaustion of caring. But some women, particularly older women, used to their husbands being 'in charge' of the major decisions, may find taking over that role late in life rather daunting.

'He had always done all our financial arrangements, and I realised that I had entirely depended upon him in certain ways. He always drove the car and he knew his way everywhere, so when suddenly he could not remember which way to go, it came as a bit of a shock. I had to cope with a gradual handing over of the things he had always done.'

You don't stop being a wife or husband or son or daughter or loving friend when you find that you're caring for someone. You're still whoever you were before, and probably just as caring as you ever were. The difference is that you simply become even more important than you were, and that's how you should regard the term 'carer'. To be 'someone who cares' is wonderful, and you should wear the term as a badge of pride.

How you approach the caring role will depend on who you are looking after. Caring for a wife is not the same as caring for a mother, and caring for a husband is very different from looking after a father. They will have different expectations and different comfort zones, and whether you're a loving wife or husband, a caring son or daughter, or a warm-hearted friend, your role will depend on your relationship with the person with dementia. If you're caring for a parent, there can be an uncomfortable point where the parent–child roles seem curiously reversed. That shift is easier to handle if you can force yourself to rise above the sadness and treat it as a chance to care for someone who cared for you as a child. Caring for a spouse means a gradual shift towards sharing responsibilities, before the inevitable and lonely point where that develops into taking over the decisions.

Yvonne sighs as she thinks about how her husband has altered since the first signs of memory loss and confusion began to trouble him. Her love for him is still very much there, but the nature of her feelings has changed. He still makes physical advances to her, and she can only gently push him away, and that's something they are simply unable to discuss.

'That wonderful, tall man that I married has become so childlike. He used to be quite a fiery person and he has become such a gentle, grateful soul who loves me lots, I do know that. But things like going to the loo have become very tricky – he can't remember how to do his trousers up. So now I am in a "mothering" role.'

'For better or for worse.' That's what the small print in the marriage service says. But an experienced GP sometimes advises her patients who are caring for a spouse with dementia to try viewing it as a new start, a completely new relationship built on showing love for someone whom they have loved and cared for over the years.

'They're not the same person they were before. I think if you spend the whole time being upset that this is not the husband you married, it's simply heartbreaking. So if you can think, "This is someone I've cared for in the past who needs my care as a nurse, as a caring person," that sometimes makes it easier. Otherwise it can be just unbearable.'

teamwork

'Happy families are all alike; every unhappy family is unhappy in its own way.' This famous line from Tolstoy's novel *Anna Karenina* could be rewritten for the dementia age, as every family will approach caring for someone with dementia in a different way – but the people who work as a team are often those who give the best care.

The dynamics of each family will dictate which family member will take up the main caring role. Often it will come down to who is still living in or nearest to the family home, who has some experience of caring, or who has most 'free' time, and there may be an automatic assumption that the bulk of the care will be done by the women of the family.

Between husband and wife there's an expectation that one will care for the other, but the carer–spouse will still need support from other members of the family. If one family member feels lumbered with the caring role, then that can quickly lead to terrible resentment. And if there is no surviving spouse to care for the parent with dementia, for example, there's certainly no agreement that dumps all the care load on the unmarried daughter, or whichever child has settled nearest to the family home.

> **'My sister could help with her car. I know she's busy and she's got a son to look after, and my brother has got his family. But just because I'm the single one and have lived near Mum and Dad all this time and looked after them, it doesn't mean that I inherit all of this. If I had a family what would they do then? They've got to do their share as well.'**

Rebecca believes that her brother and sister simply had no idea what she was coping with every day caring for her mother, until she became so stressed that she booked a four-day break for herself, and they had to take over the daily caring routine.

> 'That was the first time that they could actually see what I had to contend with, because she was getting very confused by then. The first text I got from my brother was: "Oh my God, I'm going to end up in a mental home!" ... and that was on the first day!'

Whatever your feeling about who should be the main carer, caring works best where the responsibility is shared and no one person is left to absorb all the stress of the day-to-day care. If you've seen the nature films of penguins surviving snowstorms in the bleakest windswept landscapes by taking it in turns to stand on the outside of a group huddle, enduring the worst of the cold before they yield their snow-battered place to another, then you will know that penguins can teach humans a lot about burden sharing.

How you apply your penguin-derived learning will depend on your particular circumstances, but whether the person with dementia is a spouse or partner, a parent, a sibling or a friend, the advice is always the same – build the best team you can find. Talk to everyone in the family and include them in discussions about how each one can give the person with dementia the best support according to their individual strengths and circumstances. And go beyond the family. Overcome any natural reluctance to ask friends for help by considering how bad you would feel if one of your friends was in the same position and felt unable to ask you for help. Whether it's friends or family you bring on to the team, share out the roles according to people's strengths. Some will work best when given a specific regular task, like spending time chatting to the person with dementia, or going on a walk together, so that the main carer can have a few hours to regroup. Others may have perfect shoulders to cry on, or will be happy to contribute in other ways, perhaps by researching the care options, filling in long and turgid forms or being set loose to deal with officialdom.

'My brother would have taken on the worry and the responsibility, but he's the sort of person who gets into a flap, so that's why I ended up taking the lead role in caring for Dad. My brother would know that I'd get certain things done, and I'd respect him for the strengths that he has, like always keeping people positive and cheerful – they just love him in the care home.'

All relationships in families are complex and different, and some will slide more easily into the caring role than others. But even where someone feels unable to join in the hands-on caring – whether it's just unwillingness to see the changes in a loved one or because of past difficulties between family members – stay in touch. It's important for all family members to realise they can make a difference by keeping in contact and helping in their own way.

'My older sister never had the same relationship with Dad that I managed to have, but because she's got a well-paid job, she is happy to pay for things that he needs. She has always said, "You do the caring, and I'll pay," and she only sees him a few times a year.'

When one parent has dementia and the children have dispersed and made new lives far away from the family home, it's much harder for them to be part of the caring network. That's when numbers will count, as each person's contribution – although small on its own – can build up into a useful support package for the caring parent, and opinions can be checked and feelings shared, as Lynne found when she and her brothers were supporting their father.

'I think having three of us was wonderful. The difficulty was the distance between each of us and our parents. I was the closest, about an hour away, but I had a busy job and a family to look after. Keeping in touch through email was fantastic, so we could agree who was doing what and divide up the responsibilities, which made it much easier.'

Being part of a team means that you have some support to bolster you when things get tough, and sharing the good times will help you all through the bad times. But not everyone will join in and want to work with you. Stephen was surprised that his wife's brother just refused to take any part in her care when she developed dementia, even though they had been close. He kept the brother informed, hoping he would change his mind and visit them, but eventually admitted defeat.

'I've said to him I won't get him involved in it. I will look after her, and that's it. It would be nice to be able to talk to him about it, but I think he just doesn't want to understand. He's not at all empathetic about how it feels to her.'

Stephen's support comes from their children and from local friends, but he can share the frustrations and counter some of the stress by talking to his sister. Although she lives too far away to help with the actual care, she is a good listener when things have gone badly.

'She is really, really supportive in that emotional sense. I phoned her the other night, when I'd really mucked up and my wife was in tears, and it helped just to hear her say, "You're going to get it wrong sometimes." She was able to put it all into perspective for me.'

Sometimes others in the family may resent the amount of time you spend caring for your loved one, and that can be very awkward to handle. Jane is sad that her son was just too young to get to know her mother as a fun-filled granny before the dementia changed her into someone who needs care and competes for her attention.

'As far as he's concerned, my mother is just this rather irritating old woman who takes me away from him. Every weekend I spend one day with her, and I think that's difficult for him to accept. I rarely take him along because it's not fair on him, and all I can do is explain that I feel about my mum the way he feels about me.'

The situation can become painfully complex when a step-family is involved, and children from previous marriages and ex-wives want to get involved in care decisions. When Stuart's father became aggressive and needed more care and support than his exhausted mother could provide, they found a care home nearby and went through the heartache of moving him out and settling him into the new surroundings. What they hadn't expected was abusive letters and threats of legal action from his first family, upset at what they saw as his cruel abandonment. Matters took a turn for the worse when they went into the care home, were aggressive towards members of staff and took him away with them for several days.

'What made me more angry than anything was that it wasn't for his benefit. The key for an Alzheimer's patient is routine. When you take him out of a settled routine and put him in a strange place, you're just making things more difficult for him, and I felt it was purely selfish.'

In the end, Stuart and his step-siblings took the sting out of the conflict by accepting that they needed to work together to get the best care for their father. They agreed to avoid a clash at the home by letting each other know when they wanted to visit, and the 'horrendous tension' between the two families was eased.

Tensions can also arise between family members if they feel that the person with dementia is confiding in one person and excluding others, or playing Chinese whispers in recounting one carer's comments to another. Neil is glad that he and his brother have always been open and clear with each other about how they should care for their mother.

> **'There are times when Mum tries to come between my brother and me, but we decided right at the start that she might be playing these tricks. There were quite a few occasions when she said something to one of us that undermined the other one. So I support my brother, even if I don't necessarily agree with him on everything, because I can see that she is trying to get a wedge in between us.'**

He knows that their mother is getting better care because he and his brother can share their tensions and guide each other through the most awkward decisions. That's the benefit of working together.

'I do worry about my son being in my position because he's an only child. It just makes such a difference to have somebody supporting, to share the load.'

a different truth

Sherlock Holmes was fond of saying that whatever remained after the impossible explanations had been eliminated must be the truth, however improbable it might seem to be. A distorted version of this logic sometimes leads people with dementia off down some interesting and slippery pathways, when their efforts to make sense of a situation start with an incomplete set of facts, which then taints whatever deductions they subsequently make.

Imagine this sequence of events: somebody puts a key on the table, then leaves the room; you put the key in a cupboard to keep it safe, and leave the room; the first person returns and asks you what you've done with the key. With all those facts at hand, your answer is clear. But if your memory of the third event – the bright idea to put the key somewhere safer – is missing, then the only possible explanation is that someone else must have taken the key and you are the innocent victim of a false accusation.

Of course, this is not confined to people with dementia, and it's only a matter of time before 'jumping to conclusions' is recognised as an Olympic sport. When we grapple briefly with a complicated set of data, we are often tempted to rub two facts together to spark an instant result. Reports of scientific research are frequent offenders, often noting a correlation between two statistics without proving how they are related or whether one is actually causing the other. Chocolate addicts, informed that nations with the highest per capita consumption of chocolate have more Nobel prizewinners per head of population, will gleefully unwrap another bar and draft an acceptance speech without wondering if there is a missing connection, such as the economic buoyancy of the countries or some other 'confounding variable'.

The official term for this tendency in dementia is confabulation. It is something that Graham, a GP in a large urban practice, encounters frequently in his consultations with patients who are living with dementia.

> **'Confabulation is when you don't have the right information, for whatever reason, and so you have to make up a reality that "works". People with dementia confabulate all the time. They will say that their book "must have been stolen" by somebody, because they have no other palatable explanation for it. They can't work it out or remember what happened, so they will accuse others – family members or carers or anyone – of having done all sorts of things. It's just making an acceptable and credible reality out of the bits that they do know.'**

Although confabulation is simply the innocent result of being faced with an incomplete version of events and deducing the missing part, it seems particularly common when the alternative explanation – the version rejected as 'impossible' – would mean acknowledging that they had done something unsafe or unwise, something that would increase their feeling of being out of control. To accept that they could have taken their tablets three times instead of once is in this sense 'not possible'. They are not lying; they are 'reasoning' that as tripling their medication is something they 'would never do' – and they have absolutely no recollection of having done it – it is therefore not something that they 'could have done'.

This confabulation can be very hard on the people living with and caring for someone with dementia, who can feel very hurt when the confabulated version of events points the finger at them for hiding or stealing or breaking something in the house. Graham often has to find time to talk to the relatives about their loved one's failing memory, and how the dementia might be distorting perceptions of reality.

'One patient's father had started doing this confabulation, and she was very upset about it all. But after I talked to her about it and explained that her father wasn't being deceitful and hadn't turned into a liar, she understood that it was the only way he could explain things. She felt so much better, and agreed to explain it to the family. Sometimes just allowing people to understand is enough to help them cope, rather than struggling with a father who seems to have turned into an irritable liar.'

When the person with dementia broods on an incident, this confabulation can cross over into paranoia, as an unacceptable truth is garbled and warped to shift the blame on to someone else. Before she was persuaded to give up driving, Gary's mother had a minor road accident, and the woman whose car she had driven into was very kind and helpful at the scene of the crash.

> 'My father was there, and he said that she seemed like a nurse and was very understanding about what had happened. But within a few days, in my mother's mind, all the facts had changed and she had started to believe that this woman had deliberately tried to kill her. And I don't think she quite lost her memory of that woman until she died – I presume because she had been so frightened at the impact of the accident.'

Once relatives and carers have understood the basis of confabulation – that it's caused by poor data, not by malice – it's much easier to work with it, rather than meeting it head on. Directly challenging a confabulated version of events is not going to shift a view that has been rationally built on faulty foundations.

> 'What you learn as you go on is that there's just no point in criticising people with dementia who confabulate, because they don't realise they've done it, and so they will just feel they're being unreasonably attacked.'

everyday care

Stride boldly into a stranger's kitchen – your mission is to make a cup of tea. Regard all the smooth surfaces, the expanse of cupboards with identical glossy doors concealing whatever delights are stored there ... because this is your chance to play 'Guess which cupboard contains the teabags'. Scrabble at a few false drawer fronts in search of a spoon and wonder why the fridge is disguised as another cupboard.

Experts agree that people with dementia should be cared for in their own home for as long as possible, but there comes a time when their homes need to be made more suitable for them to live in comfortably and safely. Carers and family members will need to look at rooms and household items with a critical eye, taking into account how perceptions and cognitive patterns change with dementia. Simple tasks that people have performed without much conscious thought can become strangely long and convoluted procedures in the middle stages of dementia, and they are likely to need help and understanding to carry on with everyday tasks as the disease progresses.

Take the kitchen as an example. A tidy kitchen with everything tucked neatly away may be a source of great pride and joy, but to someone with dementia it can seem a bleak landscape shorn of clues as to where to find whatever they might need.

'A friend went on a dementia awareness session and they asked him to write down in detail the steps you need to go through to make a cup of tea. Of course, the first step was to get a cup ... Well, where are they? In the cupboard. Yes, but which cupboard?'

One way of signposting and putting function first is by replacing the solid doors on kitchen units and cupboards with glass-fronted doors. This can instantly translate a series of uniform and anonymous doors into a friendly guide to the contents of each cupboard. Alternatively, placing the ingredients for making comforting warm drinks – teabags, coffee, cocoa and sugar – in transparent storage jars on the work surface will have the same effect. A mug tree or hooks to hang mugs where they can be seen will help make the whole process much more straightforward.

You might prefer other ways of clarifying where things are and what they're for. Simply putting a large label on the important cupboards is one strategy, but some people with dementia will resent this and find it humiliating. If you're looking for crafty solutions, try asking the children or grandchildren to make a beautiful colourful drawing of, for example, a steaming cup of tea for the cupboard where the mugs and teabags are kept, and a big tin of beans for the food cupboard. One partner even labelled key objects around the house with their names in Italian and English, claiming that it helped him brush up on his language skills.

Once you've found the cup and the teabag, how user-friendly is the kettle? Some kettles are designed so that it is easy to see how much water they hold, while others guard their contents like a commercial secret. Malcolm and his wife had always enjoyed sitting down together with a nice warm drink, but he became an expert at jumping up to put the kettle on before his wife offered to do it.

> **'I eventually had to stop her making tea or coffee because she kept boiling the kettle with no water in it. I suppose the upside of that was that I no longer got coffee so strong you could stand a spoon up in it or tea made of nothing but hot water and milk.'**

The downside was that his wife felt another black mark was made against her name, another despairingly simple task added to the list of things she couldn't do. It is possible to find a kettle that is easier to use correctly, so that the important sharing of the tea-making chore can continue. Finding one with a clear indication of how much water is inside is a start, but the switches on kettles also vary widely – the simplest types for people with dementia to use have a large visible switch that clearly shows when it's been switched on, either by a button lighting up or by a clear shift in the position of the switch. Some kettles, with tiny switches tucked away, are much more confusing.

Just replacing a kettle or any kitchen appliance is not straightforward in a household affected by dementia, where the advantage of buying something designed to be easier to use can be outweighed by the challenge for someone with dementia of coping with unfamiliarity. If you can't find a new kettle that works just like the old model, then it may be better to stay with the old one until you are forced to replace it. It's a problem that frustrated Patrick, as he wondered what he could do to help his wife carry on playing an active role in the house.

> **'We changed from a gas cooker to an electric one because having gas seemed to me to be much more dangerous for her. And then she couldn't use the electric cooker because it was all new and confusing.'**

Changes that Patrick began to introduce around the house to allow his wife to carry on as normal an existence as possible seemed to baffle her more, with the result that he became exasperated and she felt even more helpless and confused.

> **'It became more and more obvious that she was simply unable to work out how to use any of the new equipment that I was buying, unless the new item operated in exactly the same way as whatever it replaced. So the timer on the new cooker was "stupid", the new remote control for the TV was "unusable", finding stations on the radio by her bed was "impossible" – anything that I changed seemed to disorientate her.'**

His wife had always done the cooking, leaving Patrick in charge of the garden, but the jobs she had done in and around the kitchen for years with hardly a thought became bewildering and complex procedures that she could just not get right. Food was forgotten, shopping half done, meals undercooked or blackened, and saucepans boiled dry as the basic steps of cooking were jumbled in her mind.

> **'If you're cooking some potatoes, you've got to find the pan, you've got to add the right amount of water – and the potatoes! And then you've got to turn on the electricity or the gas – there's a lot to remember! Most of the time we just laughed at the result, but sometimes there was a bit of shouting.'**

If there's no need to change the standard household appliances, then it makes sense to keep the ones that the person with dementia has become familiar with. Newer models are often more complicated, and many carers looking for a replacement washing machine, for example, will wish that manufacturers did not provide a dozen different washing cycles to perplex confused users.

Sometimes carers can head off confusion by foreseeing the difficulties that could prevent someone with dementia from feeling able to carry on with everyday tasks and pleasures. As you know that short-term memory retention becomes erratic in dementia – particularly in Alzheimer's – then try to imagine how you can help your loved one retain as much independence as possible in the early stages.

> **'There's no point in being cross because she has forgotten someone's birthday or forgotten a hair appointment if she doesn't know what day it is. She may remember the appointment, but she can't get to the hairdresser if she doesn't know that it's Tuesday.'**

So carers can achieve great things simply by having a clear calendar or large diary on display in a prominent place, one that makes the current day and date very obvious. Perhaps you can build in a ritual of crossing off days as they go by, so that today is always highlighted. That can be enough to prod recall of some events in the early stages. Higher-tech solutions can be forbidding to set up, but a well-chosen digital calendar–clock can even flash up important appointments as a helpful reminder.

A new piece of technology that several carers have found wonderful is the digital photo frame. Once it's been set up to show a range of different photographs, they have found it a very useful tool in stimulating memories and conversation. Most have used it to show photos of friends and family members – particularly old photos that somebody has scanned; others have found that a mix of pleasing or evocative photos can also lift the mood of their loved ones.

> **'It is fantastic, because it's constantly triggering memories, which is good in terms of just keeping the brain going. And it's a constant source of conversation. If other people come into the house**

they'll start talking about the people in the photographs, or admiring the views.'

As dementia moves on and the retention of information and context becomes unreliable, you may find that simple pieces of equipment that people have lived with happily for years can start to be perceived as sinister. It's common for people to joke about not looking in the mirror too often as they get older, but a mirror can be intensely disconcerting for someone with dementia who has lost the ability to recognise the person glimpsed in shiny surfaces. If people living with dementia have gaps in their sequence of memories, and they have retreated to more secure, earlier memories of themselves, then the aged person who stares back at them from mirrors, and perhaps appears to be stalking them, is at best unsettling and at worst a threatening presence.

Some carers report real violence, as their loved ones hit out at mirrors or other reflective surfaces. The only solution if this happens is to remove or obscure the mirrors. Bathroom cabinets with mirrored doors are a major problem, because people with dementia rightly feel more threatened by what they might perceive as an intruder or stalker in that intimate setting. Covering the mirror with a friendly picture or material will prevent them feeling unsafe and upset.

Telephones can also hold a hidden menace for people with dementia, especially when they are trying to conceal the fear that their cognitive powers are declining and are treating those around them with suspicion. When a carer is talking on the phone, the other half of the conversation is unheard, and that can trigger real agitation and worries that secret plans are being made.

> **'Whenever I spoke to Mum, it always had to be on the speakerphone, because she could never talk without Dad there. Somehow he knew that he would be talked about, and he insisted on hearing every word. Now and then she would pretend to look for something in the car or the garage, so that she could talk openly to me for a few minutes and tell me what was really going on.'**

Talking on the telephone becomes a challenge if your short-term memory lets you down. The back and forth of a conversation becomes particularly confusing when there's nobody in front of you and no visual clues, so people with dementia lose track of who they're talking to or what has been said. Carers often find that their loved ones are increasingly reluctant to use the phone, fearing they might suddenly find themselves stranded, fumbling for the context and feeling way out of their depth in a phone call they cannot understand.

> **'Using the telephone has become a big problem – in fact, he just won't pick it up any more when it rings. Talking when there's nobody in front of him is difficult, because his short-term memory has gone.'**

It's not only conversation that is undermined by the loss of short-term memory. Whatever just happened is a central part of what is currently around us, and what is about to happen. The data that goes missing from that working space of the brain is the foundation and explanation of the immediate future, and losing track of it makes everyday life gradually less comprehensible. Keeping track of the twists and turns of what's going on in the cinema, for example, becomes exasperating, as Geoffrey found when attempting to preserve the 'normality' that he and his wife had enjoyed before her dementia.

'Whenever we went to a film, she couldn't follow the story, so she said every film was "awful" and we left – I never saw the end of the films. She had a particular dislike of violence in films, so we couldn't watch thrillers or any film without a simple storyline. And the same went for most of the programmes on TV.'

Nobody could fault Geoffrey for wishing to hold on to the relationship that he had with his wife, but he came to accept that if they were going to enjoy their time together, then life would have to be different. Like films, television becomes more confusing in the middle stages of dementia. Programmes that they used to regard as fun, entertaining and fast-moving may become a blur of noise and flashing lights for people with dementia, and drama or thrillers with a complex structure and large cast can be far too difficult for someone without short-term recall to follow.

> 'He just sat in front of the television watching sport because that was all he could watch. At that stage he couldn't watch any programme where there was conversation because he couldn't follow it. Sport was safe and simple, because it was just people knocking a ball around.'

Some programmes may remain watchable – carers give examples of their loved ones still watching wildlife documentaries, sport or even children's television – if they can be enjoyed 'in the moment'. People with dementia can benefit more from watching things they enjoy together with a loving carer than from struggling with more difficult shows.

As the person with dementia loses the ability to concentrate and feels more restless inside, carers tend to find that more and more activities become disrupted. Both Geoffrey and his wife used to enjoy reading, but as her mind lost the ability to focus on the developing story, she lost interest in it, and became impatient with Geoffrey's continuing interest in books, from which she felt excluded.

> 'She'd tell me we don't want to sit here reading … and she wouldn't let me use the computer because she couldn't understand what I was doing.'

The continuing march of dementia will dictate how long you can carry on with activities you love, and when you will need to find new distractions and interests to provide stimulation.

'You find things that work – whether your person is still at home or in care – and you continue with them until they don't work ... and then you ditch them. You don't go on pushing ideas or activities that have stopped being useful, because the illness has just moved on.'

CHAPTER 5

common concerns

aggression

A satirist once described a dog as aggressive because it defended itself when it was under attack. It's a description that could be applied to some people with dementia, as they battle against the shifting shapes that delude and distress them more and more. For carers, buffeted every day by the demands of caring, to be on the receiving end of aggression from their loved one can feel like adding insult to the emotional injuries they already carry, and for some it can be the final straw.

Enid cared for her husband for years as dementia slowly consumed him, feeling almost shut away with him and the disease but driven on by steadfast love and loyalty. She found his increasingly distrustful and hostile attitude towards her very hard to cope with, even though she knew it was caused by the dementia and was completely out of character for the man she loved. As his imagination took hold of him and he seemed to live in his nightmares, a growing aggression towards his wife emerged.

'He began to be suspicious of everything I was doing, and I got the blame for everything. All I was doing was caring for him, but he would accuse me of going out in the middle of the night, and he believed there were tunnels under the floor, and lifts, and goodness knows what.'

Scott noticed the same deterioration in his mother's treatment of his father as he cared for her at home, and he became concerned that the hostility she started to express was adding intense stress to the already draining task of caring for her.

'The dementia brought out characteristics in her which were there before but which had been fine. She had always been forceful, very articulate and very clever, but she became more aggressive and more paranoid – and much more intimidating.'

The aggression can develop at any stage of dementia, but it is more common in the later stages, although different forms of dementia unfold in different ways. People who have fronto-temporal dementia often undergo radical changes in their behaviour towards others, rushing in where they would normally have trodden more carefully. The crumbling of their inhibitions may also unleash unrestrained sexual behaviours that are very disturbing to all around them, and they may respond with aggression or even violence to any interventions or attempts to control them.

In cases of vascular dementia and dementia with Lewy bodies – both these types of dementia are known to generate hallucinations – although the aggression is directed at the carer, it may in fact be intended to ward off imagined threats or be set off by an imaginary situation.

With Alzheimer's disease, as in all dementias, the aggression may be triggered by fears – of what is happening to them, or of surroundings or people that they no longer recognise – or by frustrations at their inability to get things done or to communicate how they feel.

Some older men, who may have been in a dominant role all their lives, find it unsettling and challenging when they no longer feel in charge either of themselves or of the world around them. Veronica's husband had always been a self-assured man, used to taking the lead in his professional life as well as at home, and he now bristles and struggles to accept the change of roles that his vascular dementia is forcing on him.

'As the dementia has progressed it seems to intensify that assertive side of his personality. There aren't significant personality changes but there's much more frustration and anger, and it's very much directed at me. If he's reading the paper and I'm getting on with things all is fine, but once a problem arises, no matter how tiny, he gets extremely angry.'

The first rule in responding to aggression is don't respond but this simple rule can be desperately tricky to put into practice, especially when your nerves are raw and you're boiling over with exactly the same fears and irritations as the person ranting and raging at you. There in front of you is someone you care for who is ungratefully and unreasonably shouting at you, after all you've done ... but that's not what's really going on under the surface. Take a slow, long breath and look again, and you can see someone you love who's terrified or lost or tormented – probably all three – and who just doesn't know what to do except howl. Never has your help been needed so desperately, and yet it's not easy to give that help when you're so anguished and tense, as Judith found when her husband's exasperations exploded.

'It's frightening and you feel very vulnerable. The truth is you don't know whether it's personal or not, and it's such a big thing to deal with. Over time you have to learn not to take it personally, but at the beginning it is a really difficult emotional period.'

The immediate priority is to restore a sense of peaceful balance, and your best chance of achieving this is by not retorting and giving the person with dementia space. Try to regard the situation with detachment. Don't take the aggression personally, but view it instead as a possible indication of pain, sadness, discomfort or embarrassment. See if gentle reassurance or some simple distraction will defuse the tension and re-establish some calm. You may find you're so tense that the best thing is to leave the room, and, if that is a safe option, it's a much better choice than trying to have the last word and fuelling the frustrations. One carer, who somehow upset his wife first thing in the morning, was very pleased to discover that the best remedy was usually to retreat from her anger and then to return several minutes later for a completely fresh start, by which time she had usually forgotten the previous botched attempt.

Once you've managed to cool things down, take a moment to analyse what might have sparked off the aggression, so that you can work around it in the future. It can help to think of aggression as a general signal that some need of the person with dementia is not being met. Common triggers include feelings of embarrassment, humiliation or fear, but the outburst might also be triggered by pain, a sudden noise if there are too many people around, or the irritation of being criticised when everything seems to be against them. Sometimes it's difficult to put your finger on a single factor, and it is often just a build-up of general frustration at the way things have turned out. This is, of course, the hardest to predict and work around.

Sometimes the aggression goes further than verbal outbursts, and you may need more than just self-control and tact on your side. Phil finds the violent eruptions very upsetting, especially when his father's temper suddenly flares up out of nowhere.

'I was visiting a while ago and it was all fine for two to three hours and then he suddenly threw a plate of sandwiches at me. He's tried to attack me and tried to punch me, but he's slower nowadays.'

When the aggression crosses the line and turns into real physical violence, carers have to make sure they protect themselves – this is a serious and overriding priority. Discuss your fears with your GP and the community mental-health team – they may be able to recommend something as straightforward as a change in medication – and if you feel there is a real threat, you should make that very clear.

Louise feels that the worst side of her husband's dementia is his anger and the aggression that he sometimes displays towards her. His temper burst out when they were with a group of friends on one occasion and they were taken aback at how hostile he was.

> **'One person there happened to be a psychiatrist, and she took me aside and told me that I could not continue to look after him if he carried on behaving like that.'**

He would wake in the middle of the night in a fury and scream at Louise, and in one four-hour daytime rage he chased her around the house, forcing her to hide in the garden and call for help. The antipsychotic drug he was given as a result made him worse – paranoid fears that shadowy people were after him drove him to hide knives in his bed, and Louise had to put a lock on her bedroom door – until by chance she met a neurologist who advised her to review his medication with their GP.

You should ensure that you have a safe place to go when violence flares up, as Bridget found out when her husband got agitated one night. He ended up in the middle of the road shouting at traffic, and she had to call an ambulance. Once the paramedics had given him a sedative and put him back to bed, they told Bridget to call again if she needed any more help, and she went to get some sleep in a separate room.

'But the sedative wore off, and about an hour and a half later, he was up and shouting, getting really angry. I locked myself in and he was banging on the door and screaming, but I had left my mobile phone charging downstairs. This went on for a couple of hours, and then it went quiet – and by then I was so exhausted that I just went to sleep.'

The more tired and exhausted the carer and the person with dementia become, the more chance there is of one of these distressing incidents occurring – and they become more likely and more distressing at night. Partners find it particularly difficult to treat the person whom they have loved for years as someone who might harm them – it can feel like an unforgivable betrayal of someone you may have shared your life with. Understandably, partners may need others – neighbours, friends and children – to persuade them to have a safety plan just in case the situation gets too much for them – somewhere they can be safe, such as a room with a lock they can use, and a means of contacting somebody close by or the emergency services. That might mean installing another telephone extension, or buying a cordless phone or a mobile phone.

In care homes, the staff try to take the occasional burst of physical aggression in their stride. Visiting her father one day, Heather was waiting for the lift and she exchanged greetings with 'a sweet old man' standing nearby. When the lift door opened, her father came out and shook his fist in the other man's face, gruffly telling Heather not to talk to him.

'The staff told me that the two of them had had a big scuffle at breakfast that morning. I was all apologetic about it, saying it was so out of character for him, but they were quite relaxed. They told me not to worry as they'd be best friends again by the next day, and they said that the women are much worse!'

Dampening down a disagreement during daylight hours in a care home with professional staff around is very different from facing aggression when you're on your own at home in the middle of the night. For Bridget, a frail woman in her 80s, the fear of violence from her own husband brought with it the realisation that she had perhaps done all she could do for him and he now needed more help than she could provide.

'He had been up during the night and had got dressed – I'm not sure he had got into bed at all that night. I can't remember what time it was, but I woke and became aware that he was up. I looked into his bedroom and was starting to go in, but when he saw me there was a very strange look in his eyes. He came towards me and started physically to push me out, so I closed the door and wondered what to do next. And that's when I thought: this is it, I simply can't do this any more.'

clinginess

In basketball there's a defence tactic called a full-court press. Each defending player shadows a member of the opposing team, dogging their every move like a deranged stalker wherever they go on the court. It's a physically draining style of play, which has been described by one coach as '40 minutes of hell'. That level of exhaustion is not uncommon among carers of people with dementia, particularly when the person with dementia is unwilling to let the carer out of his or her sight. The 'clinging' stage is one of the times when the act of caring can become a gruelling ordeal.

After the shock of realising her mother had dementia, and the changes they had to make over the first year or two, Terry remembers how concerned she became about her father, who was the sole carer. He was completely devoted to looking after his wife, but she clung to him all the time, never allowing him a moment's break.

'He was quite clearly bearing the brunt of all this. He was being woken up through the night. She wouldn't let him use his computer at all, and she wouldn't ever let him speak on the phone unless she was right there, listening to every word. So I began to feel she had made him a prisoner.'

Very similar anxieties were experienced by Roy and his siblings. Their father seemed suspicious that they would all plot something against him if he let them out of his sight, and they could all see how frazzled their mother was becoming.

'We would try to be there every weekend, even though we all lived at a distance, just to give our mother some respite. Dad would never allow us to talk to her alone, but at least if we sat with him, she could go and have a doze. In fact, she was so drained by it all that she wasn't capable of much conversation.'

As he cared for his wife through this clinging stage, Geoff's father was largely forsaken by their friends. He was desperate to get out of the house, so he arranged for them both to visit Geoff for some lunch and a bit of fresh air, and Geoff found it almost impossible to get his father on his own.

'After lunch I would try and get my son to stay with Mum for a few minutes so I could talk to Dad and find out how things really were. But in the end he pleaded with me never to leave him with her again, because as soon as we were out of sight she would start to panic and ask where Dad was.'

When desperation got the better of her, Terry consulted a specialist in geriatric care about her mother's stifling dependence on her father, which was seriously threatening both his health and his sanity. The specialist's advice was to try to understand what was going on in her mother's mind by thinking of her not as a malign presence, but as a toddler. He explained that the social niceties that govern our behaviour are one of the last layers to form as children develop, and some forms of dementia appear to strip them away first.

'Toddlers are constantly holding on to their mum's skirt, they are terrified when their mum leaves the room and they don't like changes in routine. They feel the world revolves around them, and they have no social niceties, so when they want something, they want it now – and when they don't like something, they just won't have it!'

The 'toddler' behaviour described by the specialist – and noted by many carers – shows signs of what developmental psychologists call 'insecure-resistant' attachment. This is a phase that is characterised by extreme distress when the main carer is absent, which may turn to anger when they return. It became a painfully familiar scenario for Jacky, who felt under siege as her husband became more and more insecure and demanding.

'He got terribly panicked whenever he was left on his own. He didn't really have any sense of time. I went out of the room once for literally two

minutes, and when I came back he thought he had been on his own for hours and hours, completely abandoned.'

Experts suggest that the fear and insecurity in children can be reduced when the carer is calm and lovingly available. Tackling the clinginess in people with dementia can follow the same lines, but the situation can sometimes be prevented by introducing other short-term carers on to the scene as early and as naturally as possible. Blending in outside help early in the process – and before you get to the stage of desperately needing it – may be an effective way to prevent that clinging dependence on the main carer from developing. Of course, it's not simple if the person with dementia resents that intrusion, as many do. You may choose to use subterfuge to sidestep that problem by, for example, introducing the extra carer as a friend or a cleaner.

Where you're dealing with one of your parents, you may even encounter resistance from the other parent. Kim and her brother persuaded their father to bring in a professional carer quite early, just to be there and help around the house. But one day after leaving her and his wife alone while he took a break, he suddenly fired her.

'When he came back, Mum had gone crazy with him. She knew what was happening, so she told him that this woman was appalling and that she had been rude to her. So my dad fired her! But of course she was really a very nice woman, and then the agency

wouldn't deal with my dad any more because he'd got so cross with one of their best people.'

What upsets Kim and others is that nobody was able to advise them of the trouble ahead if they allowed their loved one with dementia to become totally dependent on a single carer. Paula's mother also wanted to care for her husband in the best way possible, but Paula feels that the result was bad for both of them as they excluded everyone else. Neither one of them could cope with anyone else joining in with the care, and if her mother had also become ill, then caring for her father would have been desperately difficult.

'I really don't know what Dad would have done without her. And if he hadn't died, I don't know how much longer she could have carried on. Her face was just grey by the end. She'd be up with him all through the night, and then she couldn't face leaving him in the day.'

As people with dementia thrive on routine – possibly to offset the turbulence and confusion they feel inside – the smartest move is to introduce other people into the caring circle as early as you can. People who are accustomed to having an 'open house' where friends and family are frequent visitors tend to find this easier than those who live a more secluded life. Try introducing potential relief carers as friends who've dropped in for tea, or as someone who shares an interest or hobby with the person with dementia. Find out about your local day centre and see how your loved one handles a few hours in a different environment.

A little perseverance is often needed to override initial reluctance, but if you succeed, the reward will be a degree of flexibility in your care arrangements and you will let some space and fresh air into what can become a stifling one-on-one relationship. Beverley's husband clung desperately to her day and night during his last year with dementia, and Beverley feels that the unbroken 24-hour intensity of the final months made it much harder for her to cope when he died.

> 'It is so much worse than a "normal" death when you've been glued to the person and you cannot leave him for a second. Somehow when they are gone, the void is even greater – it must be like losing a child.'

sleep

Being deprived of sleep – which the poet Wordsworth described as 'the mother of fresh thoughts and joyous health' – is known to make people irritable and less focused. In fact, the effects of not getting enough sleep go much deeper than that. Research has shown that it can have similar effects on your reasoning powers and reaction times as levels of blood alcohol that would cause you to fail a breathalyser test.

What is the relevance of this to dementia and care? Well, although the phrase 'sleeping like a baby' doesn't ring true to many parents, our sleep patterns do gradually deteriorate as we get older. A typical healthy 30-year-old shows a much tidier sleep pattern when monitored through the night than a healthy 65-year-old, who will usually show some signs of restlessness and disrupted sleep. When the sleep–wake cycle of someone with dementia is mapped out in the same way, the disruption is noticeably worse than someone of the same age who doesn't have dementia. Tracking the wakefulness of an octogenarian with advanced dementia is likely to show that the normal day–night cycle of waking and sleeping has completely collapsed, with sleep bleeding into the daylight hours and agitated wakefulness invading the night.

That natural sleep-wake cycle – commonly known as the circadian rhythm – is kept in sync with the actual 24-hour cycle by the sequence of light and darkness, which resets our internal rhythm (usually slightly out of sync) like a watch that is always running slow. This is key to maintaining a healthy sleep pattern for everyone, and particularly individuals at risk of disrupted sleep. Sleep researchers argue that without exposure to a clear cycle of light and dark to keep our sleep patterns on track, our internal clocks soon begin to drift and our sleep becomes increasingly fragmented, as Judy noted of her father.

> **'We did have terrible issues with the time and with his sleep. He would see a clock saying four o'clock and he'd think it was four in the morning. And, even though it was broad daylight outside, he would be wanting to go to bed. He became completely disorientated like that.'**

The scientists who first analysed sleep did not come up with inspiring names for the five phases they identified. In Stage 1 we drift in and out of very light sleep, and are easily disturbed, sometimes waking ourselves with a sudden muscle spasm that feels like falling. Stage 2 is a slightly deeper phase, measurable by the gradual slowing of brain waves, which wind down further as we move into the deeper sleep typical of Stage 3 and the deepest sleep in Stage 4. Stage 5 – the REM (rapid eye movement) stage – is unique to mammals and is characterised by rapid and irregular breathing, a faster heart rate and raised blood pressure. You may have seen this stage in a sleeping cat, its rest lit up by slight twitching movements, impulses fluttering through its body as though it was skimming through a training film on catching mice.

Experts describe REM sleep as a deeply restorative phase that appears to stimulate and renew areas of the brain that are associated with learning and memory. But they are still discovering an enormous amount about what is actually happening in our brains during sleep. With improved scanning technology, neurologists have been able to measure the activity of individual neurons in a sleeping brain, and have found persistent activity in the entorhinal cortex, a bridge between the 'old' and 'new' parts of the brain that is associated with the processing of memories. Lack of REM sleep has been found to inhibit the process of consolidating our memories of what has been learnt, more than interference with the non-REM stages of sleep.

When sleep is disrupted, we know that life seems tougher and our bodies don't work well, but chronic sleep deprivation can be toxic, weakening the immune system by depleting the number and vigour of the white blood cells that fight off infection in our bodies. Rats deprived of sleep died within weeks as their immune systems surrendered, and a review of sleep research in humans concluded that regularly sleeping for less than six hours a night could lead to serious health consequences. People in one study who woke frequently during the night were found to be five times more likely to have amyloid plaques (see page 20) in their brains than those who slept well through the night. Other research showed that levels of the protein beta-amyloid – a key component of the plaques found in brains with Alzheimer's disease – were higher in mice during waking periods and lower when they were asleep. The plaques formed more quickly when the normal sleep cycle was disrupted.

A classic problem in the middle to late stages of dementia is the 'sundowner', the person with dementia whose natural sleep–wake cycle is disrupted to the extent that dozing during the day becomes the norm, which can lead to disturbed nights full of restless wandering around the house. And carers, faced with exhausting physical and emotional demands on them throughout the day, rely more and more on being able to recharge at night.

So what advice can help smooth out sleep problems? For people with dementia, what they do during the day can lead to much calmer nights. Increased exposure to natural bright light during daylight hours will help their inner clock keep better time, and physical exercise and just keeping busy will also prepare the way for a quieter night, according to an expert.

> **'If you can get out in the morning for your exercise and have a walk, that will be the most effective thing that you can possibly do – in terms of light exposure, morning light is the most important.'**

This doesn't mean it has to be an expedition with a big stick and bagfuls of Kendal mint cake. Just parking a little further from the post office, or strolling around the park to feed the ducks is likely to have a positive effect. If you can make it a pleasurable ritual that the carer and the person with dementia enjoy together, you can both benefit from the shared exercise and change of scene. Even just resting on a bench when you've walked enough will still count – it's the brightness of the light outside flooding into the eyes that does the job. As we grow older, our eyes require more light for everyday tasks than they did when we were reading teen magazines, due to physical changes in the eyes – the pupils become smaller and the lenses thicken and become yellower and more opaque. Even on a cloudy British day, when light levels outdoors may limp up towards a few thousand lux, that may well be ten times higher than the light inside the home. On days when you're unable to get outside, siting your loved one's favourite chair by the brightest window and raising the normal indoor lighting levels through the day can help stabilise the internal biological clock and reinforce proper sleep timings.

This is just as important in care homes. The light levels in some institutions for the elderly have been measured at a ludicrous, torpor-inducing 20 lux during the day – that is comparable to the night-time lighting of main roads. A small-scale study in the Netherlands has shown that installing brighter lighting in the living areas of a care home has positive effects on both restoring the sleep cycles and raising the cognitive awareness of residents.

Just as higher levels of light during the day will help restore the daytime rhythm, so lower light levels and a more tranquil atmosphere as you approach bedtime will help trigger a sleep response. Keeping to a routine of relaxation is also likely to help you lead a loved one towards sleep – perhaps do the same gentle activity every day, such as listening to music, looking through photographs or having a calming warm drink. Through trial and error you will discover which activity your loved one finds most soothing. Rachel realised that their bedtime routine was more straightforward when she allowed her husband to get himself to bed in his own meandering way.

> 'Getting to bed at night, it was much easier if I came away and let him get on with it – he'd get there eventually. But if I stayed in the room with him, nothing would get done: he'd just wander busily around. So I would just leave him to it, knowing he would get to bed, and I would go to bed to get some sleep.'

And what advice for carers, for whom sleep is a vital regeneration of energy? However bad it gets, don't believe in the effectiveness of a nightcap (the strong drink sort of nightcap, not the Wee Willie Winkie type). Neurologists warn that although alcohol may help you drift off to sleep, it actually disturbs the deepest levels of sleep, including the valuable REM sleep. It is far better to try to find your own relaxing rhythm – it may be a comforting warm drink, a gentle mind-walk through your favourite happy memories or an unwinding playlist on your iPod. Perhaps listen to the soundtrack of a film you love that you can 'watch' with your eyes closed, or search through bookshops or libraries to find a good audio-book so that you can lose yourself in a soothing velvety voice breathing life into a familiar story.

If you do find that your level of worry or the restlessness of your loved one is regularly preventing you from getting enough sleep, talk to your GP. Sleep disruption is one of the key triggers of the decision to move someone with dementia into a care home, because if you are short on sleep, then caring will become desperately difficult, as Rachel discovered.

'In the middle of one night I became aware that he was up again, and that's when the truth hit me: if I can't get a decent night's sleep, then I just can't do this any more.'

appearances

How many times have you been told how wrong it is to judge people by their appearance? Or that there is much more to someone than just how they look? Yet it's apparently only human to ignore that advice every day and give overriding importance to our first impressions of someone. Research reveals that the outcome of 20-minute job interviews could be predicted by analysts who viewed only the first 30 seconds of the interview, during which the interviewer and interviewee merely shook hands and sat down. They allowed no time to listen to even a single question; nothing more than a quick glance up and down, and minds were already made up.

Appearances are, of course, superficial and insubstantial. They shouldn't matter, but we know they do. There are shelves full of self-help books on how your clothes or your shoes can affect your mood and alter the way you perceive yourself. If you can help someone with dementia to look better, then it is possible that they will feel more in control and will see that others treat them with more dignity.

'My dad didn't know how to blow-dry my mum's hair. So I used to go home and I would tell her that if she would have a shower – because that was beginning to be a problem as well – then I would blow-dry her hair. In the end, when I realised how much that mattered to her – because how you look defines a lot how other people will treat you – it really was worth having Mum's hair done at the hairdresser every week.'

Nicola discovered that this decision made a huge difference. Her father was given a precious hour of freedom once a week while her mother was being pampered and having her hair done. Her mother – who had always liked to be well dressed and with her hair nicely done – was allowed to feel she was still special, and that in turn helped her father in caring for her, because it helped him to see her as the woman he loved, not as a stranger. So simply making sure that the person with dementia still looked presentable and as normal as possible was good for everyone – good for her mother and good for her father, and therefore good for Nicola, too.

Your clothes and the image you present are, particularly for women, fundamental ingredients of your self-image. They are a public statement of who you feel you are, and there comes a point in dementia when that is lost. The whole area of dressing and undressing and changing clothes becomes a battleground. The person with dementia loses the interest or ability to do it well or regularly, and the carer can quickly decide that just getting your loved one dressed is draining enough – any clothes will do when you're exhausted.

'It would take Dad about an hour to get Mum to take her clothes off to go to bed at night, and then another hour to get her out of bed and dressed in the morning.'

When the carer is a husband looking after a wife, he may well be at a loss when dealing with women's clothes. And men, fighting to preserve their independence, can be very grumpy when they feel 'nagged' about what they wear. This is a situation where Nicola feels that children or friends can really make an impact and ensure that the person with dementia doesn't look like a wreck.

'If someone can go out and buy some basic clothing, that is a great help. Just being sure that the person with dementia will be in a clean top and clean trousers matters a lot for personal dignity. I don't mean smart clothes, just fresh clothes so they get used to the idea of changing clothes. And you have to be a bit brutal about throwing old things away, because they will forget. And if you let someone look a complete mess, then everyone reacts to them in a different way.'

It's also worth looking for clothes that are tidy enough to look good, but easy enough to slip on and off without too much disruption. Many carers find that they need to consider buying larger or smaller clothes, according to how well the person with dementia is eating. Some eat less and worry more, while others put on weight as they become less mobile and perhaps forget that they've already eaten.

While you're still at the stage of keeping up some sort of normality, making sure the person with dementia looks normal and has clean clothes may be quite important. The unpleasant reaction of neighbours when his wife was brought home after an emergency stay in hospital still distresses Colin, who had taken great care in looking after her through her dementia.

'She was in a dreadful state, because she didn't recognise where she was, and she'd get scared, she just looked terrible. A neighbour had told someone in our road that "a mad woman" had

moved in, and for my wife to be called a mad woman was really upsetting. It's so insulting, so unfair, but that's how she appeared to other people who didn't know what was going on inside, what was happening to her.'

Encouraging her mother to keep to a routine of changing her clothes was certainly important for Jill, although preventing her from looking 'like a wreck' turned out to be a considerably harder task than she had expected.

'We had literally to change her underwear for her, because she couldn't or wouldn't do it any more. She'd just go to sleep in the clothes she was wearing. I tried to do it for her, but it was like trying to get clothes off a dead body because she'd stiffen up – she wouldn't allow me to undress her because I'm her daughter. She just refused to accept that she was supposed to get changed for bed, and then get changed all over again in the morning into different clothes.'

Yet there comes a point when the battle to keep the person with dementia looking as he or she always did becomes tinged with a denial of the reality. At least one experienced professional carer argues that the pressure to preserve appearances creates unnecessary tension, and feels that it's better to focus on the needs of the person with dementia, and step back from worrying about whether that top matches that bottom.

'Carers and families really struggle when loved ones stop being impeccably dressed and very clean – if they could only forget about them looking weird and stop worrying about what they are wearing. If they feel comfortable, leave them be and they will be less scared and aggressive.'

There does come a point when concentrating on the appearance of someone with dementia can become a distraction from giving proper care. A wish to keep up morale and preserve the image of your loved one is understandable, but if it means fights over clothing every day, you will have to quietly ask yourself if it really matters. People with dementia may choose scruffy and comfortable clothing to avoid having to fuss with buttons, hooks or zips that they find increasingly fiddly. Although it can be cruelly hard for the carer to accept, a more relaxed person in the 'wrong' clothes may be much more like the one you love than a smartly dressed person, cajoled into the 'right' clothes, but who is resentful and tense.

getting personal

'There are certain things I think a son doesn't want to do for his father, and we broke one of those barriers within a few weeks of him moving in with us. I was standing in the bathroom and heard myself say, "Okay Dad, you can come and put your

teeth in now ..." because I had been scrubbing them for him. And that was something I had never really planned to do.'

Caring for someone with dementia will take you on a strange journey, moving you way outside your comfort zone. As well as the emotional distress of seeing someone you love become confused and lost, you have to cope with physical needs and the hardest part is usually involved with intimate care – and it gets a lot more intimate than brushing Dad's dentures.

'There is going to be a point where Mum is going to need a lot more physical help. I don't know what I'll do then. There's a lovely walk-in shower with a big seat in it, so I hope I won't ever be at the point of showering my mother, but I suppose you can never say never. We will have to wait and see.'

In fact, many older people with dementia will stop showering or bathing, perhaps because other concerns and worries cloud their day and the thought of undressing and washing all over just seems like too much to take on. It maybe adds to the feeling that everything is falling apart.

'When I noticed that Dad was wearing the same favourite jumper every time I saw him, I confronted him and asked when he last had a shower. He would tell me that he had a shower twice a day, and would never admit he hadn't had a shower ... perhaps he really thought he had had one?'

As dementia progresses, the simple everyday act of bathing or showering – usually a time to relax and briefly bask in the physical pleasure of warm water – can become strangely disturbing. People with dementia may see the water in a bath as menacing, their perception of its depth wildly distorted, which sets off real fears of drowning. It may be the reflective surface of the rippling bathwater that sparks this panic, and you might try adjusting the light in the bathroom or adding some bubble bath that they can gently whisk around the bath before climbing in.

Some people become equally frightened of showers. It may be the confined space of a shower cubicle or the hissing noise of the running water that scares them. You may find that keeping the shower door open or the shower curtain folded back makes life easier – even though you will have to dry off the floor afterwards. Holding the shower head and directing a very gentle spray in strategic areas is often better than leaving it to splash everywhere, and calm or distracting conversation may help a person with dementia survive the ordeal.

Keeping them warm throughout the process is very important. A warm bathroom will make them feel less exposed and vulnerable as they undress, and there is true snuggly comfort in being quickly wrapped in a large warm towel or dressing gown after their bath or shower.

'My husband simply hates a shower because when I turn the shower off, he immediately feels cold – and he doesn't understand that the cold feeling goes when you put a towel around you.'

If bathing or showering the person with dementia becomes a battleground, then you may feel you need some help. Many carers turn to social services or professional carers to manage the hygiene needs of their loved ones, who often show far less resistance when somebody from outside the family takes charge. When Yvonne's husband defies her efforts to help him get washed and dressed, she gets the impression that his anger is not really aimed at her, but it still prevents her getting the task done.

> **'He'll confront me over silly little things. He'll insist he doesn't want to get up and he'll just shouts "I'm not getting up now!" So now we have a carer every morning who comes in and helps him up, gets him showered and downstairs, and he's fully cooperative with her.'**

But there is an even more awkward area to tackle, as people in the middle to late stages of dementia may also become frightened of using the toilet. For some, it's related to confusion in a claustrophobically small room, where the toilet itself may be hard to distinguish from other objects – some rooms are beautifully coordinated in the same colour, others are all dazzlingly white – especially when the seat is down, and possibly covered with a fabric cover. For others, it's a fear of the toilet itself, as Grace found with her husband, when it became impossible to persuade him to undress and sit on this strange opening down which rushing water would suddenly disappear.

'One of the things he began to find scary was the toilet. It started to feel like this strange black hole, which he was scared he might fall down. So he lost the sense of what a toilet was, and he was terrified!'

It's usually in the later stages of dementia that people tend to become incontinent, either through lack of awareness of the need to use the toilet or through confusion – perhaps feeling unsure where the toilet is, for example, or simply not moving quickly enough to get there. Like most carers, Gordon found this a very unpleasant part of looking after his wife.

'In the end she couldn't do very much for herself when I was looking after her. The real bad bit is ... it's like having a child, taking her to the loo and ... sorting her out. That was the worst part for me.'

He tried to persuade his wife to wear adult nappies to keep her dry through the night, but she would rip them off. For the last six months of caring for her at home, he was changing the sheets two or three times a night, and mopping the floor between the bed and the bathroom on those occasions when she did try to reach the toilet. By the end, he was dealing with her double incontinence.

Being prepared for this stage is essential, if you're going to carry on caring at home. You will need a mattress cover, a good supply of easily washable bedding, a reliable washing machine that can cope with washing very soiled clothes ... and an extraordinary amount of loving patience.

'I was getting up in the night, stripping her bed and putting the bedclothes and her nightclothes in the washing machine and remaking the bed. And then two hours later it would all happen again.'

Gordon's son was terribly concerned for his father's health through this stage, as he became more and more drained, resisting his children's attempts to persuade him that he had done enough and should allow others to take over the caring role.

'How he kept on doing that, night after night, I do not know. That whole incontinence thing is an absolute nightmare, and my view is that from that point you shouldn't go on caring at home because you just can't cope.'

People in the middle or later stages of dementia can also suffer from acute constipation, which may not respond to the usual laxative remedies. It's as though the brain stops responding to signals from the bowel, and the ability to 'push' seems to go. In the more serious cases it can require medical intervention, as Sammie found with her mother.

'She had always had stomach conditions, but since the dementia she's had to have three bowel excavations because she gets so constipated. Because she had dementia, she didn't know what was happening except that it was very uncomfortable and it made her very agitated

and sort of "crazy". This is what caused the twisted bowel: she's had that twice. Every time she had something like this, I was hoping that she would return to me as she had once been, but of course it never happened.'

Caring for a loved one through the sad decline of dementia can be an intensely painful process, and one of the hardest decisions to make is when to stop. Andrea, a trained carer, has seen the spouses of people with dementia making themselves ill by just carrying on and pretending they can cope with the strain.

'The elderly generation believe it's up to them to care and they are very reluctant to ask for help, often even from their own children. But it's such a big responsibility at so many levels that people just wear themselves out – they can't see what they're doing to themselves. And when people look back they can see they definitely should have asked for help earlier.'

As their loved ones progress, step by tiny step, through the stages of dementia, carers are reluctant to let them down. So they assimilate each extra little demand that is made of them, slipping gradually beyond the point where they should call for help.

Having to admit that you can do no more can feel like failure and betrayal, and carers may need a trusted friend or relative to show them how much they have done and to help them take the difficult step of recognising that they cannot go on this way. The friend will need to convince them that accepting help is not a sign of weakness – it really does require strength to acknowledge that others can help to give a loved one the best possible care.

'It was only when my wife was taken into hospital and the doctor said, "This man cannot possibly cope alone at home looking after this woman," that I was somehow able to give myself permission to ask for my wife to be taken into a care home.'

CHAPTER 6

essential techniques

humour

This may seem to be the wrong time for humour, but resist the temptation to tear this section out and stuff it in the food processor just for the joy of watching these words being ripped into a jangle of letters that more accurately reflects how you feel. Save this section for when you can find comfort here, and use the release of those oh-so-painful and oh-so-valid emotions.

The power of laughter has been known for centuries. It's around 3,000 years since Solomon observed that a merry heart did as much good as medicine, and science has gathered good evidence to support that view. While a group of volunteers were shown part of a stressful film and then part of a comedy, researchers measured the diameter of their blood vessels. The results showed that the stressful sequences caused their vessels to constrict and the funny film made them relax and dilate, with a difference in potential blood flow of 30 to 50 per cent between the constricted and dilated states. As the lead researcher is reported to have said afterwards, prescriptions for good health should include laughter.

Perhaps that explains why people in stressful situations – such as the carers of people with dementia – have sometimes found that seeing the funny side of otherwise upsetting incidents in the middle of their labours can be genuinely helpful. Philip's father is in the middle stage of dementia and living with him and his wife in a self-contained granny flat. Although his behaviour can be very strange, the occasional joy of shared laughter reminds Philip periodically that the real 'him' is still there inside.

> **'Most weeks there are glimmers of who my dad was – sometimes they're only obvious to me because I'm his son and we have that sort of bond. Every so often he will say something, and cackle ... and I'll think, "That's my dad!" And we'll just look at each other and laugh, like we always used to do. So he is still that person, for that one brief moment.'**

Sometimes humour can emerge from the place you least expect, and that's part of its delightfully subversive power. Sian recalls how her mother, who had been rather stiffly domineering when bringing her up, spent an afternoon taking great delight in the sort of earthy potty humour that she would never have tolerated before dementia changed her viewpoint.

'When my son was about eight or nine, we used to go and see Mum, and it must have been terribly boring for him. Well, as he was sitting on the sofa next to her on one visit, he discovered that he could make "farting" noises with his hands. A few years earlier she would probably have told him off, but she loved it and just giggled every time he did it. And they were so happy together, farting away on the sofa for quite a while.'

Edward would occasionally think it was odd that he rarely got any post, and he tended to blame the postman. It wasn't until they were moving house that he found that his wife had hidden several bin bags full of letters behind the sofa, perhaps fearful of what they might contain. Tom never had to ask his mother if she was still using the car, because he noticed that a parking ticket would arrive each time – until she finally gave up driving.

Humour can take many forms, but it's sometimes a release of tension – a way of coping with an awkward or emotional situation. When circumstances face you with the choice of laughing or crying, there isn't a wrong choice. Either response can bring release in its own way, and both are equally valid reactions, but laughter is usually more enjoyable. Incidents that frustrate you or make you sad may be seen as funny later when the passage of time has smoothed the raw edges.

Carol was able to see humour at the end of an exhausting but apparently wasted day – although she must have wished that she could share the joke with her dad. Worrying that he was not really looking after himself properly, she used to prepare a batch of meals for him, arrange to take a day off work and organise a friend to pick up her children from school. After trundling down the motorway, she would spend a busy day sorting things out with him, taking him shopping, tidying up the house and then leaving him a list of all his favourite food that she had put in the freezer before joining the crowds on the way back home.

> 'And then when I got in there'd be maybe 10 messages from him on the answerphone, all saying, "Oh, I thought you were coming down today." So I'd pick up the phone, rather grumpily, and remind him that I had already been down, and he would say, "Oh, that's a shame. I must have missed you." And when I told him to look at the food I had put in the freezer, he'd just say, "Oh, I must have gone shopping after all ..." And so my whole busy day would just have been wiped out of his mind.'

As their memories falter, people with dementia can offer innocent amusement to their loved ones as their food-related habits float free of long-held convictions about what they enjoy and what they would never ever eat.

> 'Dad never used to eat chips – he would always say he didn't like chips but, once he had forgotten that he didn't like them, he would eat chips very happily!'

Steven also described how he had taken his father out from his care home to a smart restaurant – the sort where a waiter hovers around constantly offering bread rolls. During the meal, he had become concerned at how hungry his father was.

> 'I watched as Dad would go through five or six bread rolls. At first I was worried that he had not been getting enough food in the home, and then I realised that he had simply forgotten that he had already had two or three or four rolls.'

For Richard's mother, every meal can be a wondrous plateful of surprises, because however often she's enjoyed the same food before, the tastes can ambush her anew. If he ignores the repetition, and simply savours her repeated delight at what is put in front of her, their mealtimes can be full of smiles.

> 'Everything is new to her – it's wonderful. So every time we have yogurt, she says, "Oh, this is lovely!" and she carefully makes a note to buy some the next time she goes out shopping.'

Other everyday household problems may be tackled in unfamiliar ways. Knowing there was no washing powder at home, George picked some up while he was out shopping. He was then surprised to see all the laundry hanging up to dry when he got home.

'I was wondering how my wife had managed to wash them, and then I saw the green splodges all over the white sheets. She'd put over three-quarters of a bottle of washing-up liquid into the washing machine. We did four more washes without having to put any more washing stuff in.'

When your wife goes out for a walk, the last thing you expect is to see her carried home like a pharaoh, so it was a sight that brought a smile to a worried Robert. He and his wife used to try to fit in a short walk every day, but their plans were often thwarted because she would be distracted, or take ages to choose the right shoes, or she might suddenly decide that she needed a sleep instead. One day, Robert had already started cooking by the time she finally declared herself to be ready, so she said she was going to go without him.

'She didn't come back for quite a long time, and eventually I thought I'd better go and see what was going on. So I went out and found this procession coming towards me. Apparently she had fallen over, and had been lying on the ground – quite contented – until these people found her and fetched a chair for her to sit on. And then she insisted that they had to carry her back in the chair. So there she was, issuing orders magnificently as four of them carried her in state on this kitchen chair.'

Amanda managed to use the humour of a situation to defuse her mother's anger when she was detained in a hospital's psychiatric ward, where her treatment made her very cross. Amanda was sitting with her mother when a nurse came over to check her, but the nurse saw she had a visitor and said she'd leave her in peace for the time being.

> 'Then Mum suddenly said, "Bugger off! I don't care if I never see you again!" Normally, of course, I'd have said something like, "That wasn't very nice, she's only doing her job," but instead I joined in and agreed with her, saying how terrible that nurse was. Then my mum started to laugh, because she was no longer the angry one. Suddenly we were both together in the "bugger off!" club, and she was all smiles.'

Even when they're being put through the distressing indignity of having their cognitive skills measured, people on the borderline between mild cognitive impairment and dementia can still find humour in their situation. Sandra was using the MMSE test (see pages 55–6) to assess one elderly gentleman in her surgery, and was at the stage of testing his awareness of the world around him. He was spot on when asked what year it was, and she then quizzed him on the date.

> 'He considered this for a moment and said, "It's February, doctor. It's February the fifth." Well, I thought that was fantastic, because he'd struggled a bit on some of the other questions, so I told him

> he'd done really well on that. And he smiled at me and said, "Thank you, doctor. You know there's a calendar on the wall just behind you, don't you?" So there's a lovely example of someone who has a bad memory but still has perfectly good cognitive skills.'

Psychologists looking at stress and successful coping strategies have demonstrated that people whose sense of humour was rated as high on something called a multidimensional sense of humour scale showed fewer signs of stress and reported feeling less anxious than those whose sense of humour was rated as lower than the norm. Their findings reinforced the belief that 'seeing the funny side' really can be effective in taking the sting out of intensely difficult experiences. There's a mental flexibility – like a tree that bends in a storm, rather than snapping – in seeing both the tragedy and the comedy of a situation. Finding the humour in predicaments that would otherwise be unrelentingly grim has been shown to work as a 'coping strategy' by helping to distance people from the stress.

Caring for someone you love who is struggling with dementia can easily drop you into stressful situations that you would not wish on anybody, and where a sense of humour mixed with some loving detachment may be your only hope of coming out sane. When Julie called in after work one day to see her mother, she was complaining of an upset stomach and said rather suddenly that she needed to use the toilet. Rather confused in her urgency, she couldn't find the right room so when she did get there with Julie's help it was too late. In a moment they were both standing in a pool of her mother's diarrhoea, and Julie was wondering what on earth she was going to do – and wishing she could just disappear.

'Then my mother suddenly turned to me and said, "Who has made this disgusting mess?" Well, I couldn't think what to say to her. If I told her that she had done it, she would be furious and say she would never do that sort of thing. I could try telling her that John had come in from next door and done it while we were downstairs, but she wouldn't like that much either. I really didn't know what to say, but I suddenly realised that there was only one thing that she needed to hear. So I said, "Mum, I don't know ... I really don't know who made this mess, but I promise that when I find out who did it, I'm going to give them a piece of my mind." And she held my hand and said, "Oh, thank you, darling" ... And that was it!'

Of course, there was still the mess to clear up. Seeing things through a filter of gentle humour and understanding didn't clear that away, but it did save Julie from making a mess of her relationship with her mother – and that was a triumph.

change your mind

Changing your view of events around you can have an extraordinary effect. A recent review by public health experts of more than 200 studies concluded that the way you look at the world can have a serious direct effect on your health. The research showed that people with higher levels of optimism and happiness had a reduced risk of heart disease and stroke. But the effect of looking at things in a positive light can be more immediate – simply changing the way you think about a problem really does change how you tackle it and how you feel about it. All you have done is to change the approach in your mind – and those who cannot change their minds cannot change anything – but that can literally transform the situation.

After years of hard work, Laura's husband retired and they both looked forward to relaxing and spending time travelling. But she soon discovered that his vagueness and confusion, which he had shrugged off as 'just a bit of stress', were in fact more serious symptoms of dementia, and their plans had to be shelved. The disappointment could have felled Laura, but she faced the setback with a positive attitude.

> **'I decided very early on that wherever he is in this dementia spectrum, it's the best it's going to be, and I should make the best of it. And I think that's really important. I can't just sit there and think, "Oh, this is terrible!" …'**

By refusing to see their situation as a tragedy, she feels more in control and is able to take real pleasure in ensuring that he gets the best care that she can give, and she knows that she is only doing what he would have done for her. Their everyday life changes as the dementia moves on, but she keeps her husband and herself in good spirits.

'You certainly need to keep a sense of humour when you're dealing with something like this. When funny things happen, I do laugh about it – and I laugh about it with him, too.'

Researchers who have found that optimists enjoy better health and live longer than pessimists have speculated that people who habitually look on the bright side are better at coping with adversity when things do go wrong. Like humour, optimism builds resilience, and gives you the strength to tackle problems that would floor a pessimist. Winston Churchill, not a stranger to difficult situations or dark thoughts, was a fan of optimism: 'A pessimist sees the difficulty in every opportunity; an optimist sees the opportunity in every difficulty.'

You may find that some well-intentioned people confuse 'looking on the bright side' with 'ignoring the sad truth', as though crooner Bing Crosby was right when he equated accentuating the positive with eliminating the negative. Lorraine winces when her friends seem to coo at her and gloss over her husband's difficulties, now that his dementia has left him confused and passive.

'I find people are always telling me, "Oh, he is much better today!" or "He's not so bad, is he?" It's almost like they're reassuring themselves and that doesn't give me much leeway to say, "Well, I know

he was fine when you came, but you should have seen him half an hour earlier," without sounding all crabby.'

Looking for positive aspects does not mean closing your eyes to the sadness. The bad parts of caring for someone with dementia cannot be avoided, but focusing on and emphasising the good parts, and realising how they can be an unexpected source of strength, can give carers the chance to enjoy those moments that they are still able to share with their loved ones. Clive's wife had always loved gardens, and one of the last pleasurable activities they shared was a visit to a National Trust garden.

'She loved it. She started to tell me how her grandmother used to take her there in the late 1930s. She was recounting how the gardens and the trees were then, and how it had all changed. As she was telling me, she forgot who I was, she was back with her grandmother. It was beautiful ...'

Patricia had similar positive experiences in the later stages of her mother's dementia. She had always been a rather cold and controlling parent, and Patricia feels she might have remembered her with some resentment if the dementia had not taken away her domineering aspects, and imposed a kinder softness on her.

'One thing I found extraordinary was how she reverted to her childhood, and remembered the

> **most amazing things that she had never told me before. It was almost as if her memory for those days was coming alive again – and that was rather lovely, particularly when you got her talking about it.'**

Perhaps some people work on their ability to keep a positive attitude in the face of caring for someone with dementia. Perhaps they have a special gene that helps them regard going upstairs and forgetting why you went up as an invitation to do it again, and enjoy the extra exercise to boost the cardiovascular system and enhance brain power. Maybe they can even see the repetitive questions of someone with dementia as a chance to find the right response, like the character in the film *Groundhog Day* who is condemned to repeat the same day until he gets it right. Or perhaps those people are just following Winston Churchill, who explained why he was an optimist by saying: 'I am an optimist – it does not seem to be much use to be anything else.'

music

When all around you is turning to dust, where can you obtain a feel-good substance in safe doses that will – briefly, safely and at no charge – lift you out of the ditch and gently smooth out the wrinkles of your soul? Look around you – there is probably a dispenser of this wonderful stuff near you right now.

Now that you no longer need to employ a minstrel or hire a small orchestra to have music around you on demand, we have become used to it as a background noise wherever we go. The true strength of music is not in its ability to mask the clunking noises of machinery from a lift full of nervous strangers. It is that it has the power to touch people deep inside, restoring and repairing where it reaches.

Scientists have even watched the physical effects of the most passionate and emotional music, using brain scanning to analyse what goes on inside when people hear their favourite piece of music. What they discovered is that when we listen to a piece of music that sends tingles up and down our spine, the body releases a chemical called dopamine. This is a neurotransmitter popularly known as the 'feel-good' chemical, which is associated with giving us pleasurable feelings to 'reward' behaviours that have a positive value in evolutionary terms (the usual examples are eating when hungry, making love, slaking a deep thirst – all activities that benefit the survival of the species, and are therefore candidates for reinforcement). That's why a choice piece of music can reach past our emotional defences and give us a hug when we most need it.

Many people, particularly those under pressure or pinched by stress, find that music can transport them at no cost to a happy place deep inside, the same peaceful space that hypnotherapists help them find when dealing with buried fears and worries. Whatever your taste, from Meatloaf to Mantovani, Sting to Stockhausen, allowing a few minutes to suffuse yourself in the music that touches you really can give you a lift and ease your tensions.

Music also speaks to people with dementia, and can communicate so much to them without making any demands, although many find continuous background music both distracting and unsettling. Most effective, as they move into the middle stages of dementia and right through into the later stages, is music they recall from their happiest days, which often stays alive inside them together with the feelings that the music first sparked in them. Charles Darwin noted over a century ago how 'the sensations and ideas excited in us by music ... appear ... like mental reversions to the emotions and thoughts of a long-lost age'.

Although your neighbours may wish it wasn't true, the effect of music can be even more powerful if you join in and sing – it may be the benefit of breathing deeply or the sheer emotional release of singing, but serenading your radio while the kettle boils or livening up a traffic jam by dueting with your favourite CD can help lift the greyest of moods. If you enjoy singing with others, the positive feeling can be more than doubled by joining a choir. Don't be afraid of having to go through an audition – many choirs value enthusiasm above proven ability and you will learn as you sing. Somewhere nearby you are sure to find a local choir that would welcome you. For example, the British Choirs on the Net website (at www.choirs.org.uk) lists more than 3,000 choirs, catering for all sorts of musical tastes and abilities, and groups singing in the rock or glee styles are popping up in towns all over Britain.

Kath encountered the reviving power of song while visiting her mother in her care home. During a lull in conversation, she started to sing a song she'd heard her mother enjoy – 'If You Were the Only Girl in the World'. In a moment, she became aware of a little old man dragging himself over towards her and her mother from his seat on the far side of the room.

> **'One of the carers brought him a chair so he could sit in front of me, and the eye contact with him was amazing. My mum and I were holding hands and singing as this man joined in, and he knew the words far better than I did. At the end of the song, he grasped my hand and said, "You're a diamond!" still staring deep into my eyes.'**

On subsequent visits, he showed no signs of recognising Kath until she began to sing with her mother. Then, like a battered old chair coming to life, he would grind into action, get up and shuffle over to be part of the music-making again. The staff told Kath that he hardly ever spoke and spent most of his time sunk in his chair, but when he heard the old songs it was as though fairy dust had been sprinkled on him. He rose up, his face animated and his movements determined, showing the power of music to reach out to somebody through the deepest channels when other systems of communication appear to be shut down. (Scientists will suggest that this is because the right anterior temporal lobe – where neuroscientists believe we store our musical memories – is not significantly damaged by Alzheimer's disease, but it remains a joy to see!)

And if you don't enjoy singing, then get moving. Roger and his wife had always loved the music of the dance bands that had entertained them when they were young. When his wife developed dementia, Roger was sure their dancing days were over, until a friend suggested that it might be the perfect tonic for her.

'He found a few places where they do dance sessions for people with dementia. It was lovely. These people are sitting there, almost lifeless, until the music starts, and then they're up on their feet, some of them dancing beautifully.'

It's not easy to get much done when you're dancing, but a small-scale study in Sweden recently tested the effects of mixing a little singing into the morning washing and dressing routines of people with severe dementia. The results showed that they were much calmer and responded better when their carers sang, and this was accompanied by a marked drop in cursing and aggression, which supported the findings of other studies on the benefits of music in caring contexts. The authors of the Swedish study also noted that musical therapeutic care requires nothing more than the carer's voice and minimal training, yet can achieve similar effects to medication without the risk of side effects.

Organised activities involving music are particularly popular in care homes, and many put on special musical events, either featuring professional performers or singalong sessions focusing on well-known songs – the favourites are popular songs from the 1940s and 1950s and Christmas carols.

'The musical afternoons are wonderful, although the effects can be so short-lived, because of the memory problems. And some of them don't get what's going on. But music has links that go so far back ... and people's memories for the words of these songs are amazing.'

Your loved one doesn't have to be living in a care home to take part in similar activities. The Alzheimer's Society runs local 'Singing for the Brain' sessions, which combine the power of singing with a friendly and fun social atmosphere for people with dementia and their carers (similar groups are available in Scotland through Alzheimer Scotland). Gentle warm-up exercises relax tensions and a greeting song pulls everyone into the circle. Some sessions include simple actions but the emphasis is always on joyous participation rather than potential as a soloist. As Darwin also commented, 'We can concentrate greater intensity of feeling in a single musical note than in pages of writing' – although he did wait until the 320th page of his book to make that observation.

calm and unruffled

Those of you who are already perfect can skip this section. These words will only make sense to people who recognise, firstly, that perfection is a glorious ideal that you may catch glimpses of during your lifetime if you are very lucky; and, secondly, that trying your hardest to get things right while being honest enough to admit when you're wrong and brave enough to learn from your mistakes is a lot more constructive than going all out for perfection. Insisting on perfection and then damning yourself when you fail to attain it only benefits the mail-order suppliers of sackcloth and ashes, and it does no good to you or the one you're caring for.

Imagine you are writing an advertisement for the ideal carer to look after somebody dear to you who is being ravaged by dementia. Think of the qualities you would demand to ensure the proper loving care. Very high on that list would be the ability to stay calm, caring and unruffled in the face of whatever screaming frustrations might be thrown the carer's way. Patience and understanding are the twin lubricants that can help you to override the lurching gear changes of dementia as you give the best care you can.

One deeply felt regret has been prominent among the carers who have kindly given up time to be interviewed for this book. Pauline's view is typical. Deep down she knows that she has cared for her husband as well as she can, and there's only one aspect that still bothers her.

> 'What upsets me is remembering how cross I have sometimes got with him. I want everyone to understand that they should please try to have as much patience as possible with people who have dementia, because they don't realise what's happening. They will get angry with you and start shouting at you, and you just have to let it wash over you, because they don't know they're doing it.'

Anthony is also troubled by knowing he allowed the frustrations of caring for his wife through her dementia to burst out from time to time, and wishes he had understood more about dementia and what to expect.

'People with dementia can be terribly difficult, and you can lose your rag quite easily if you're not careful. There have been times when she was so tiresome, and I used to get a bit cross with her, but if I'd known that she couldn't help it, then I think that would have made it easier for both of us.'

Learning not to react with anger can be cruelly difficult, and may go against every well-founded instinct to defend your dignity or stand up for the truth. There might be hidden resentments between you and the person with dementia, or between you and other family members, which will be like dry leaves waiting for a spark to catch fire. Even in a family where all is sweetness and light, the sapping drip, drip of endless repetition can be enough to wind up the most balanced carer, as GP Sandra acknowledges.

'In one brief 10-minute consultation, I can ignore the fact that someone with dementia will ask me the same question seven times. But just imagine what it must be like to live with that all day every day!'

Paul is one of those carers who does live with it every day as he looks after his mother. A friend of his marvelled at how he responded in exactly the same calm tone of voice however many times his mother made the same comment or asked the same question, instead of screaming, 'We've just had this conversation!' as his friend said she would.

> 'But the truth is that I don't think she would – and I don't think people in general would do that either. I have this belief that people rise to the occasion.'

So how has he learnt to live with the repetition and the frustration – or perhaps he has learnt to look beyond it? Is it simply because Paul is perfect?

> 'To be honest, it's purely self-protective. If I did react like that, I'd upset Mum, and then that would upset all of us. I know the repetition will last 10 minutes or so, and if I just stay calm, then she will move on to something else.'

So there you are. You don't even have to be perfect to get it perfectly right – just stay calm.

contented dementia

> 'I knew his wife had been diagnosed with Alzheimer's, just like my husband. He told me that she kept on wondering where her mother was, so I asked him how he dealt with that. "I tell her she's

just being stupid," he said. "Her mother died years and years ago, for goodness sake!" And I thought to myself: no, you're mad, that won't do any good.'

One of the hallmarks of Alzheimer's disease that can differentiate it from other forms of dementia is how it interferes with the proper functioning of a person's memory. Recall of recent events is lost first, while memories of more distant times persist for longer. Compare the deterioration to the gradual erosion of a landscape savaged by harsh weather. The first layers to fragment and be blown away are the most recently formed ones on top, which in turn exposes the next layers – and on it goes. Some individual events or periods of time seem to endure, isolated from any context as the surrounding memories are washed away, and people in the middle stages of dementia will cling with growing intensity to those surviving outcrops of memory.

When people with dementia lose their hold on the reality around them and retreat to the security of the past, carers often feel that a barrier rises up between them and their loved one. If their partner or parent is lost in another era, how can they continue to communicate? Some carers – like the woman above – cannot see beyond the totally rational and understandable view that the only solution is to pull the person with dementia back into the present, as if she was resetting a watch to the correct time. Others seem to realise instinctively that it is futile to correct someone with dementia who is trying to make sense of 'today' from a viewpoint that may be trapped in a time decades ago.

Judging someone's actions without understanding their perspective is flawed from the start. Imagine someone seeing a cyclist suddenly leap off his bike and start a manic dance, ducking and twisting with wild and frantic gesticulations. The viewer's instant common-sense appraisal of that behaviour would probably involve the words 'epileptic' or 'psychotic'. Without the information that the cyclist was being attacked by a wasp, the onlooker's view of his 'dance' would be hopelessly inaccurate. Even if there were no wasp, and the cyclist was reacting to a buzzing that fanned his fear of being stung, that judgement would still be irrelevant and unhelpful. As a reaction to a wasp – real or imagined – the 'dance' is understandable, and the confusion arises only because the onlooker is not seeing the situation from the other's viewpoint.

Complaining to a neighbour about the trials of caring for his wife, who had dementia and was more and more confused about everyday living, was the catalyst for Norman's conversion. The neighbour showed him a newspaper cutting that proposed a different approach and offered an analogy to explain what was happening inside the heads of people with dementia when the 'now' around them grew blurred and they took refuge in older, sharper memories. The article mentioned a book, *Contented Dementia*, and within two days Norman had read it twice and – for the first time in years – he felt he understood his wife's behaviour.

'I remember thinking, "Yes, yes, yes, this makes sense at last!" ... and I still thank the people behind this insight every day.'

After desperate months of trying to 'fix' his wife's 'mistakes', Norman had found an alternative way of thinking that he described as a 'lifesaver'. At the heart of this approach, drawn up by a carer who spent an enormous amount of time looking after her mother through Alzheimer's disease, is a way of seeing the effects of dementia from the point of view of the person who has lost the ability to remember new events and to access certain memories. So rather than point out the errors of fact – things she has forgotten, people she no longer recognises, or confusion about date, time or place – Norman learnt that he could reduce his wife's distress and ease her tension by not opposing her as someone who knows better than she does, but by working in partnership with her.

'When my wife says, "Right, let's go!" the most natural thing for me to say is, "Where to?" or "What do you want to do?" or 'Why are you saying that?" But now I understand that won't help, because she won't know the answer and would just look at me, and we would be miles apart. But if I say, "That's a good idea," then we're on the same side.'

The approach that Norman and others have found so useful is called the SPECAL (Specialised Early Care for Alzheimer's) method, now incorporated in the work of the Contented Dementia Trust. It explains the primary problem faced by someone with dementia as a lack of information, rather than a breakdown in reasoning power. It uses the analogy of a photograph album to represent memory, with the memories of individual events as photographs stored in the album. We are continually making reference in our everyday lives to the 'photographs' of previous events – what we did yesterday, who lent us £5 or where we parked the car. But people with dementia randomly and intermittently store a 'blank' photograph, which contains the emotions linked to events or experiences but without the associated facts of what happened. Feelings become increasingly important to people with dementia; and although feeling happy without knowing why can be good, feeling anxious or distressed with no trace of where such a negative feeling has come from can be horribly unsettling and hard to deal with. Skilfully ensuring that people with dementia stay in the calmer and safer waters of good memories is the essence of the SPECAL method.

The staff in the first care home that Amanda found for her mother insisted that she took 'calming' medication because she was disrupting other residents. Amanda was convinced that the drugs made her worse – they slurred her speech and made her look 'zoned out', but they did nothing to take away her feelings of distress. So when Amanda discovered SPECAL's behavioural approach, she realised that there was a more benign way of settling her mother's agitation.

'I don't think my mum would be alive without that discovery, because I would have given in to what was being suggested, strong drugs and having her "sectioned" – they would have worn me down and I would have accepted that they knew best. But I realised we could actually sort this out

ourselves. I'm not saying it's not exhausting or terribly, terribly sad ... but at least there has been a way through it.'

She saw the method in action after her mother had been treated in hospital for an infection, and a friend who had done a SPECAL course came with her to help get her ready to come out. A defensive and apparently cantankerous woman was transformed into someone quite different.

'The nurses hadn't been able to do anything with her, but within five minutes of this woman arriving, they were doing "Singing in the Rain" together, and chatting about folding the laundry and putting it in the airing cupboard. It was all very low-key and natural, it wasn't a big performance or pretending to be someone. It's just tuning in to the person, and having a chat.'

When Amanda visits her mother in her new care home, she finds herself making huge geographical shifts in her conversations with the different characters in there. For a woman who used to live in India, a brief reference to life in Delhi gives her a boost; and a quiet man who seems lost within himself will really perk up if she mentions the name of a pub in his area.

'And there was another woman who used to walk the corridors very anxiously, asking where she could get the bus to her home town. So I would say,

"Let's see if we can find it together," and I'd walk up and down with her a few times until something else distracted her. So I have to be ready to go all over the place when I am in the home.'

There's far more to Contented Dementia's SPECAL method than just dropping in place names like a stand-up comedian struggling to bond with an audience. The whole framework can build a protective cocoon around the person with dementia. The idea is to develop 'themes' based on that person's pre-dementia life. Skilful use of those themes allows a carer to head off the agitation and wandering that can be sparked off when the person with dementia is suddenly faced by an unsettling 'blank' in the photograph album. The system also builds in an acceptable reason for the carer to be absent from time to time – often a very upsetting experience for someone with dementia – and even encourages the carer to take up a new challenge in preparation for when their caring duties will come to an end.

The SPECAL method has passionate admirers who value the simple tools it provides, but it is not without critics. Look up SPECAL or Contented Dementia Trust on the Alzheimer's Society website and you will find a rejection of the Trust's framework as 'controlling and prescriptive'. Drawing on its huge experience, the Alzheimer's Society takes the view that SPECAL is incompatible with the need to give people with dementia personal choice and control or influence over decisions being made about them – as enshrined in the National Dementia Declaration drawn up by the Dementia Action

Alliance, a grouping of more than 100 organisations. It also suggests that 'prohibiting the asking of direct questions' disempowers people with dementia in a way that may be contrary to the goals of the Mental Capacity Act 2005. However, the Society also notes that the SPECAL method is popular with some carers and includes elements that reflect established good practice; and it praises its 'emphasis on the feelings and emotions of people with dementia' as a strength.

Read both sides of the argument and make up your own mind. Only you as a carer can decide what you want to take from the various strategies on offer. Many carers adopt a 'pick-and-mix' tactic in the early stages as they search for whatever works for them and their loved one, and there can be true relief when they find their solution.

> 'What SPECAL has given me is the understanding that she is still the same person inside – and that is something to celebrate. It has helped me make my peace with her before she goes.'

caring for the carer

> 'Amongst all carers, the carers of people with dementia are one of the most vulnerable, suffering from high levels of burden and mental distress, depression, guilt and psychological problems.'
>
> Dementia 2010 report, produced by Oxford University's Health Economics Research Centre for Alzheimer's Research UK.

Caring for anyone with a terminal disease is exhausting and distressing, but when that person is emotionally important to you, someone you've known intimately for years, the distress is multiplied. If the person with dementia is clearly in distress, yet rejecting your help through fear, denial or confusion – and perhaps even changing from time to time into a hostile and aggressive stranger – the effect on a carer's morale can be devastating.

An American study of nearly 2,500 married people has indicated that looking after a spouse with dementia may seriously increase the risk of the carer also developing dementia. Working over 12 years in an area renowned for the longevity of the residents, the researchers found a 'real and persistent' decline in memory performance and cognitive abilities among the married carers, findings that went beyond other short-term studies that have shown carers performing badly in tests. The American researchers concluded that people whose spouses had been diagnosed with dementia were six times more likely to develop the condition themselves, when compared with people married to someone who did not have dementia. Although the research did not pinpoint what the cause of this heightened risk might be, it was suggested that the stress of caring for a loved one was likely to be an important factor.

For many carers one of the most stressful aspects of caring is the isolation that settles on them. In the absence of a coherent and active system of support to guide carers through these emotionally turbulent times, they often feel very much left on their own.

'The frightening thing is that if you're caring for someone with dementia, you feel there is nobody out there, no support anywhere. And yet living with dementia is very demanding and incredibly draining.'

Even the tried-and-tested remedy for stress – getting away for a break to relax and spend some calm leisure time together – may be too much for people with dementia to take in their stride. Diane felt she and her husband would both benefit from a week being pampered in a hotel, but it was to be the last break they had together.

'We tried, but we had to come back after the first night because it just didn't work. It was all too strange for him: the bathroom wasn't where he was expecting it to be and the room didn't look the same when he woke up in the night, so he didn't know where he was and got upset.'

Often carers don't know where to find support or what sort of support is available, and sometimes they don't even feel able to ask friends and family for help. That might be because they feel that a disorder of the brain is slightly shameful, or it might be through a heroic but damaging loyalty, and a sense that they should cope with the problem themselves.

'My mum didn't reach out to people, because she was embarrassed by the whole thing. There was a period when she didn't want to embarrass my dad, so she put up walls to protect them both.'

Some carers will just carry on, taking one day at a time, and putting themselves under more and more pressure. Bryn, a GP with a special interest in dementia cases, discovered that one of his patients was still being cared for at home despite being completely dependent and in need of full-time supervision.

> 'She was being looked after by her husband and two sons, and her score on the tests showed she was severely impaired. They had never asked for any help, and had just accepted that this was how things were.'

Another of his patients, whose mother was in the later stages of dementia, came to the surgery with symptoms of chronic stress. She had never sought help from anyone, and was caring for her mother day and night.

> 'I asked if she could really cope with this, because I thought her needs had gone beyond that. Eventually she realised her mother would be better off in a home, but she was racked with guilt. I've had three sessions with her just dealing with the guilt, and she's finally admitted that it is the right thing to do.'

So what is the advice to be gleaned from this? Three words – ask for help. Support is available from organisations that are familiar with dementia issues, help with caring can be provided by local social-care services, and friends and family are also one of the best resources available to carers. However, none of these potentially lifesaving groups can help if you will not let them, or will not ask for help. Share your problems with the professionals because they will understand the stresses and strains you are facing and will probably have experience of positive solutions. Ask about support groups in your area. The Alzheimer's Society runs Dementia Cafés and many other services throughout England, Wales and Northern Ireland, and many carers find great comfort in talking to others and discovering that they are not alone in the difficulties they are experiencing (similar groups are available in Scotland through Alzheimer Scotland).

Try to tell your friends what is happening early on. You may find that some friends disappear, but then you will be left with a core group of friends who understand. If you need help from friends, be brave and ask. The worst that can happen is that you remain in the situation you were in before you asked. Be clear. You will find friends who want to help but are worried – worried about doing something wrong, or just worried about everything – and they may find it easier to help if you have a specific task that they can do. Believe in your friends, trust them, and share your problem so that they can help – that really is what true friends are for.

Friends can help you unpack your feelings, acknowledging them and facing up to them so that they don't dominate you. The emotions that will swamp you may be both valid and understandable, but once you've externalised them you can often see them more clearly and are able to choose which ones to run with and which to reject. Guilt and sadness can be highly toxic when stored away and repressed, but you really can tame them by talking about them and sharing.

As you wander through painful emotional landscapes, too worn out to seek anything but short-term relief, you may even lose track of why you're doing this caring – and that is when you most need a friend at hand as a benchmark and guide. A friend can tell you that you're doing the right thing, and you're doing it out of love for someone who is in truly desperate need of your help. But you also need someone whose judgement you trust who will be able to tell you when you're taking on too much and possibly damaging both yourself and the person with dementia.

What should friends do when they discover that one of their group is facing the trials of dementia? Be honest – it's much better to tell someone that you don't know what to say than to say nothing. Offer help with quiet tactful persistence. Some people still follow a social convention that they should refuse help when it's first offered, and they may feel ashamed of needing help, preferring the terrible dignity of struggling alone. If your offer of help is rejected, smile and keep the lines of communication open so that your beleaguered friend knows that you are available, that you understand and that he or she can count on your support when it is most needed.

grief

They used to call it 'time and motion', the objective study of a workflow, deconstructed and remodelled with the aim of smoothing out a manufacturing process and removing the inefficiencies. But a technique that can work wonders in speeding up the creation of plastic pencil sharpeners should not be applied as rigidly to the unreliable, twitchy emotions that control how we feel.

Nevertheless, the shifting pain of grief has been analysed, and a glance at the five broad stages of dealing with a terminal illness, as identified by a leading psychiatrist, can be a starting point in understanding some of the feelings that will flash erratically through you. The first in her list is *denial.* You try to shut out the possibility or reality that you don't want to face, disputing and challenging, demanding a second opinion. Denial is not necessarily a negative phase, it can be seen as a shock-induced 'holding pattern', or like calling for a timeout in a hectic game of basketball so you can just take a deep breath, and ponder or prepare.

Next comes *anger*, an exhausting emotion that will mercilessly drag you through hedges in its quest for answers to impossible questions. Why them? Why now? Why is there no cure? How can life be so cruel? And you may also find that you begin to harbour a smouldering resentment against others, against contemporaries who glide on, untouched by the cruelty of dementia.

The third stage is labelled *bargaining*, which describes the twists and turns inside as you try to construct a scenario where the horrible reality is taken away from you. This is where you struggle to reverse time and take a different path in the hope of a better outcome. People with a religious faith will petition their god to bargain for a less mournful ending, and others will search for alternative methods of 'buying off' this destiny.

This stage gives way to *depression*, the numbing realisation that you cannot change this fate. It's a time of regret, a period of apathy and mourning, where you may feel dazed and withdrawn. The final stage in this analysis is *acceptance*, which may signal a weary submission as you slide towards the inevitable, or just a calm detachment.

However, these stages of grief should not be seen as a calm and dignified progression. They are not separate rooms, like the structured tour through a busy palace, where the flow will carry you down this corridor, through the drawing room and into the gift shop. At first, you are just as likely to flit around and sample all these emotions (and more) like a frantic bluebottle, and there will be days when you experience all the conflicting emotions at least twice in the time it takes for your kettle to boil. And it is reasonable to believe that the person with dementia will be somewhere in the same fog. How much insight they have into what is happening will depend on how far their dementia has advanced, but it is likely that they will be dealing with their grief and fears until cognitive decline loosens their grip on such concerns.

It may sometimes appear that well-meaning friends and the caring professions are wishing to hurry you through the stages as though they are helpfully marching you out of a maze, but try to resist them calmly. They are only looking for a way to alleviate your suffering, and that's a natural human response. Even the people who say they 'know what you're going through' or those who expect you to find consolation in the crickety nonsense that so-and-so 'had a good innings' are doing their best to comfort you. And you are sure to need friends and professionals to support you through the bad days.

Be content with grieving at your own pace and in your own style. No two people grieve in the same manner or go through the blistering emotions in the same sequence. It is intensely difficult to be tolerant of others around you who may be wading through the same grief but are stuck in 'anger' when you're busily 'denying', and then daring to 'bargain' brashly when you're up to your elbows in the 'depression' stage.

Finding a way to release the emotions can be genuinely liberating. The French playwright Pierre Corneille said that grief can often be calmed by telling your story, and if you can find a sympathetic listener, you can test his theory. Recognising the upheaval inside yourself is a major step forwards, and sharing your feelings with those around you will allow them to understand you and support you. So that when you snap at a misplaced coffee cup or a forgotten appointment, they can treat you as a rational and caring person who is under enormous emotional strain, and not as a cold fish who is obsessed by the temporary GPS coordinates of crockery.

Some Brits, overtrained in the supposed benefits of 'keeping a stiff upper lip', may find that acknowledging the grief (and they might prefer to call it 'giving in' to the grief) feels wrong. But a little structured 'wallowing' can leave you feeling much more positive and determined afterwards. You could head for the midway approach by earmarking a time to indulge and 'feel' the emotions that are probably coursing through you like a dodgy kebab. Perhaps try to set aside some 'howling time'. Slotting in an hour or two on a miserable Monday or a terrible Tuesday to let go of the sadness can give you renewed energy to carry on with the caring. Getting yourself back on track is eased by setting time limits for 'letting go'.

Another way of dealing with your turbulent emotions is to grab a pen and put down on paper how you are feeling, either in the form of a diary, or an essay, or just a formless rant. The purpose of this is not to write a bestseller, but to find a way to express – to 'ex-press' is literally to squeeze out – the tensions and sadness inside you. You might end up with something you want to keep, but some people find that 'squeezing out' their bitter and hopeless thoughts on to paper has the most profound effect when they then tear them to shreds – it gives them the positive feeling of taking control of those thoughts and purging them with an 'I-can-do-better-than-this' flourish.

Beware of people who want to modulate your grief or who seem to suggest that you're doing it wrong. The stages of grief are not a map that you should follow; or are they a declaration that 'This is where ye shall go ...' The analysis should not be seen as an attempt to control or direct the journey through grief (and, yes, it is a journey, with an ending) but as a listing of what you may pass – perhaps an I-spy book of the emotional potholes and signposts that you may encounter. Don't feel constrained by the stages, but treat them as reassurance that these conflicting emotions are part of the natural grieving process.

One more thing: with dementia, the grieving process can sometimes feel different and even more intense than grieving at a death, because the slow decline of cognitive abilities and awareness can feel like a 'loss' in itself. Some carers and family members talk of 'double grieving', feeling that they 'lose' their loved one inch by inch as the dementia carries them beyond normal everyday experiences and loving communication, and then 'lose' them again at the end. But others talk of the final release of being able to grieve for the whole person, and having the chance at last to remember them at their best.

You will – and this is the hardest part to believe – find a sort of peace one day.

CHAPTER 7

care in the later stages

social care

'Get social services involved. They're the people who know what's available in your area, they'll know how things can work financially, so get them on board. Don't be fobbed off. Get the right person. Find somebody you like and talk to them.'

This was the advice that Melissa was given when caring for her mother – who was slowly sliding down the dementia spectrum – became too demanding and time-consuming for her to fit around her busy work schedule. She was concerned that her mother had stopped eating proper meals and was forgetting to take her pills, so she turned to social services for some help to allow her mother to continue to live in her own home.

'We said we wanted someone to come in every morning, just to make sure she was up, and to give her a cup of tea and some breakfast. They didn't quite get the "dementia problem", and a different person turned up every day. So one morning Mum came down and found this strange person in her kitchen and was absolutely livid, chasing her out with a walking stick.'

Melissa's mother was furious with her children for putting her in what she saw as an embarrassing position, and angry at the stigma of letting others think that she could not look after herself, so the arrangement ended. It took some time for Melissa to pluck up courage to try again, by which time her mother was becoming more and more reliant on her for everyday care. Telling her mother that it was just a check-up to ensure that the house was safe for her, she invited social services to come and assess her needs and found she was dealing with a new person who had a much more understanding attitude.

'The woman who came round was fantastic. I explained to her the bad experience we had had with different people coming in every day, and she agreed that she wouldn't want them coming into her house. She arranged for the same woman to come round every morning just to make sure that Mum was up and running ... and that probably gave us another six months' breathing space.'

All that had changed was the personnel. Melissa believes that the first person who had dealt with her was 'just irritated by the whole thing', whereas the second person she contacted was empathetic, and could see the problem from Melissa's mother's side, instead of viewing it from her desk as a task to be crossed off a long list.

The support you will get from the local social-care structure will depend to some extent on luck and geography. Even those working in social care accept that the level and standard of support can vary enormously across the country. This is partly because of differing perceptions of priority (although supporting the carers of people with dementia is now recognised almost everywhere as a key issue) and partly because of funding constraints. But local authorities have a vital role in the delivery of dementia care, as most people with dementia are cared for in their own home by a blend of informal family care and professional carers.

Local authorities are obliged to provide services to meet the needs of people who cannot care for themselves if those needs meet certain criteria, which are decided by local councils. In practice, most local authorities will offer support only when a person's needs are assessed as either substantial (such as being unable to carry out most personal care or domestic routines) or critical (such as being liable to develop significant health problems or to be seriously neglected). These action levels, and the choice of what support will be given, are both decided locally, and therefore vary from one local authority to another. You don't need a diagnosis of dementia to be eligible – it is simply a question of what care is needed, and whether the local authority can provide the care – but support will only be offered to people who pass the means-testing hurdle.

How do you start the process of asking for support? Whether you are the person with dementia, or a relative or carer, you will need to contact the Social Care or Adult Social Care team of the relevant local authority. If you are not sure which is the right local authority, either call a nearby local authority and ask for help or search on the internet – go to www.gov.uk/find-your-local-council. When you find the right department, ask for a care assessment (some councils call it a needs assessment), which will look at the circumstances of the person with dementia and the current needs for care and support. Most requests for an assessment of someone's care needs come from health professionals or relatives, according to an experienced social-care practitioner.

> **'Sometimes it's families who will phone up because they're worried that their mum can't cope. Quite a few referrals are from GPs and other health professionals, like district nurses. And sometimes it's the people themselves and in other cases it might be friends or neighbours who are worried about someone wandering, or maybe someone who lives alone who doesn't seem to be managing well.'**

Each local authority will conduct its assessments according to its own working practices, but the aim of the assessment will be to establish what degree of care and support is needed by the person with dementia. They may ask for a carer or the person with dementia to complete a self-assessment questionnaire, but the main assessment will usually take place at the person's home, because an insight into current living arrangements may be part of the evaluation. Straightforward assessments may not take much more than an hour or two, while more complicated cases may require several visits and consultations. It is always a good idea to think through the issues ahead of the assessment and decide which are most important. Sometimes you may feel you know what you need, but in other cases you will just know the problems and the professionals will design a solution.

If the assessment finds that you have needs that should be met, then a care plan will be drawn up detailing the services that are to be provided. There will also have to be a financial assessment, since the support services are means-tested. So if you have savings over a certain level – the current cut-off point is £23,500 – then you will be expected to pay a capped contribution towards the care. If you have an income, that will also be taken into account in finalising any contribution that you are expected to pay. Each authority will have different arrangements and different measures, but the overall truth is that nobody will be deprived of a service simply through inability to pay.

With the emphasis on personalising care – that means tailoring a general service to meet particular people's needs and wishes – you may be offered self-directed support. This gives you control by giving you a budget to manage. You decide on how the care is delivered. This allows you to choose who provides the care (within certain parameters) and to take responsibility for ensuring that the care is provided.

The services available will depend on local provision, but they will be aimed at giving the person with dementia whatever care and support is needed. This may take the form of professional carers to help with washing and hygiene, or someone to provide meals where the person with dementia is no longer able safely to do so.

'Local authorities can arrange services to support people with dementia, such as home care, or day services or sometimes "extra care" housing. They may also offer simple paid-for services, such as giving a carer a break, or arranging Dementia Cafés, which give people a place to go where they can meet other people in a similar position.'

Where local authorities or other bodies offer respite care by taking the person with dementia away from their home to give their carer a break, Gillian warns against the possible disruption it can cause, as she found with her husband.

'Sending my husband away from our home, even to a respite placement that he had used before, became more and more terrifying for him. And it was traumatic for me to find that when he came back he was in a worse state than when he went away. So we pushed for a replacement carer to look after him at home while I went away for a break.'

Sometimes the measures needed to allow someone with dementia to continue living independently are more fundamental, such as specialist equipment (mobility aids are among the most common) or home alterations (converting a bath to a shower, for example). Other services may include the provision of an incontinence nurse, or a supply of incontinence pads. Always ask what is available, and keep the local authority informed of any problems that may arise or new care needs that develop. Remember, they are there to help.

'It is one of our jobs to help support carers. It is done to varying extents and with varying degrees of success across the country, partly because of funding issues. But if the local authority is supporting the person that you care for, you should have a number you can call so that someone can bring up your records and get straight back into the details of your situation if circumstances change.'

It doesn't always run smoothly, of course. Barry's family was thrown into confusion when his father's dementia worsened. It was clear that he needed help, but they had no Power of Attorney and were told by the woman from social services that she would have to assess and decide on his future. Even when the emergency services had to bring his father home, and the family had found a place in a care home, she refused to budge. When no progress was made, Barry eventually demanded a meeting with the woman's manager, and it came out at the meeting that the family had been misled and their case worker – who had been given no dementia-related training – was taken off the case immediately.

'It was so hard to make the decision that he should go into care, and that it was in his interest to take him away from home and everything that he knew. But then actually to have to fight social services to be allowed to do it, only to be told at the end of it that we hadn't been given the right information was ridiculous.'

There was also confusion about whether his father would be eligible for local-authority funding if the family chose a home that was outside the county boundaries. Asking different people the same question seemed to produce different answers each time, and Barry advises families to verify the key facts with managers, to get things written down for clarity and to make a big noise whenever you want something done.

'We never really felt on top of the process. It just felt that we had to fight to get anywhere. In the end we had to threaten people with legal action, we had really to look into what we were entitled to and go in armed with that every time to get anything done. It was all very complicated and it wasn't explained properly.'

Christopher's mother cared for his father throughout his dementia, and he feared that she was going to burn herself out completely, because she saw it as her duty to do everything she could. By the late stages, he no longer worried about his father – as he was being so well cared for – but he was desperately concerned for his mother's health and sanity. He feels that the social-care services should be more pro-active in helping, rather than waiting until there's a crisis.

'There's a point at which you have to stand up and admit you're not coping – and social services do not do it for you. I think they only react when people scream. So unless you scream that everything is in meltdown, they don't bother with you. I think they can't cope with the burden, so if you have somebody like my mum, they leave her alone.'

As an ex-manager of a social-care department, Caroline is seeing things from the other side of the fence now that she is caring for her husband. Even with her experience, she finds the system confusing, and complains at the lack of clear and direct information available.

'I feel a bit disappointed that I haven't actually been given any sort of overview of the services that they might offer us. I suppose the main thing is that people are hugely overworked and their time is always limited – but time is of the essence for us, too.'

Some cautious optimism about the provision of care services is a result of the prominence now given to dementia. According to one influential social-care professional, the Prime Minister's recent Dementia Challenge campaign (run together with the Department of Health and the Alzheimer's Society) has raised the profile of dementia care quite considerably. The hope is that the publicity will change expectations and lead to enhanced training for professionals working with dementia and better care for people living with dementia. Improvements will already be noticeable in some areas, but other issues will take longer to feed through and will need a wholesale cultural shift.

'But it isn't all about money and buying more things. A lot of this is about attitudes, it's about doing things in a particular way, and it's about understanding, compassion and dignity.'

hospital

'Those two weeks in hospital just did him so much damage: being ignored, sitting in his own filth, not being fed. It's just incredible that the people there didn't have a clue what they were dealing with. What we found was that the nurses were doing more of a doctor's job, and the actual nursing care – bringing your food, taking you to the loo, the "caring" side – was being done by people without any nursing qualifications.'

Talk to anybody caring for a person with dementia, and the conversation will often turn to how poorly many hospital staff seem to understand how dementia impacts on their patients. Perhaps they just don't have the time to consider how the limited cognitive capacity of someone with mid-stage or advanced dementia can make a stay in hospital totally bewildering; or maybe the lack of understanding is because their training doesn't even touch on those problems.

When her mother went into hospital, Katie found herself defending and protecting her as she would a child. Most of the staff made little effort to engage with her mother, and they found her difficult to deal with. In the end she was moved to the psychiatric ward after she refused to let anyone near her to wash her. And instead of ensuring that she got the nutrition that she needed, the staff would plonk a packet of sandwiches next to her, which she couldn't open.

'I could easily understand how somebody in there without a relative to watch over them would go downhill fast. The nurses were running around the ward, and they told me that Mum wouldn't take the pain-relief tablets. But it says in her file that she won't take tablets, because she can't understand what they're for.'

Even though the staff were clearly under pressure, Katie finds it frustrating that they could not use a bit of ingenuity in finding a way to give her the pain relief that she needed. Pushed into the role of advocate for her mother, she tried hard to convince the staff to listen to her mother's objections and think of a cunning plan to get around them, rather than just believing she was mad and difficult. Luckily, there was one senior nurse looking after her who clearly had a better feel for what was going on in her mother's mind. She was the only one who took the trouble to address her worries and put her at her ease, and her approach made it seem so simple.

> 'When she tried getting her to take the medicine, Mum kept asking what time her father was going to be home. So this one nurse addressed this obvious concern by telling her she wasn't quite sure what time he'd be coming back that evening, and my mother opened her mouth and took the medicine.'

Katie's anger also stems from how some medical staff seemed to regard people with dementia as somehow less entitled to dignity and respect than other patients. She recalls how her mother was treated on her admission to the hospital.

> 'There were a few staff who seemed to understand and made allowances, but generally they didn't appreciate that even if somebody has dementia, they've still got feelings! They were trying to put a gown on her, and they stripped her so that she had nothing on her top, even though two male nurses were there. She was shouting, "The men! The men!" but nobody took any action until I asked for them to leave.'

Her biggest argument with the medical people is about how they view her mother. They're trained to look at the illness, which is the reason, Katie believes, that they are sometimes unable to see the person.

> 'I saw a report on her the other day by someone quite senior, which said that she had advanced dementia, which is true, and that her conversation is reduced to a series of meaningless phrases. But it's not at all meaningless! It may not always be normal, and it may not relate to what is going on around her, but it's not at all meaningless.'

When her father had to spend some time in hospital, Lesley was astonished at how quickly he seemed to lose weight. The ward staff were keeping a food diary of everything he wouldn't eat, and when she looked at the list, she asked how they were giving him the food.

> 'The nurse said they offered him a choice of meals, but as he was never sure which he wanted, they gave him whatever was left. And they would just pop it down in front of him and leave it there. I tried to explain that he couldn't make those decisions any more, and unless someone helped him, he would just forget to eat. The nurse just said, "Oh ..." and said she'd look into it.'

The one thing that Lesley hoped for when he was moved into a specialist mental-health ward was that he would be properly looked after. But after several days she found that he still hadn't been washed.

'I was told that they asked him every morning if he wanted a bath, and he said he didn't. When I suggested they could find a way to coax him into a bath, they said if he doesn't want a bath, they can't force him. It's ridiculous. He doesn't have the mental faculties to be making these decisions for himself.'

After his mother had to have two operations, Will learnt that any stay in hospital would mean an end to her stable existence at home for many weeks after she came out. The disruption of adapting to a different environment in the hospital seemed to trigger deep-seated fears, bringing all her anxieties to the surface.

'With Alzheimer's, people have a huge problem learning anything new, because their brains are just degenerating. So dealing with new experiences becomes very problematic, because they are less equipped to make any sense of them.'

Will can see a link between any traumatic experiences and deterioration. Every trauma his mother faces – such as not really understanding why she is being taken from her home and put in hospital for two days, where she is confused and frightened – marks a setback. He blames the confusion and upheaval for exposing the underlying weaknesses in her abilities, and it can take weeks or months to get her back on an even keel again.

> 'This is the second operation she's had in six months, and we've seen a big decline in her cognitive ability, in Mum's ability to cope. She's very tearful, upset and confused about where she is and who everybody is. We get her back on an even keel by just being gentle and giving her as normal a family life as we can. I'm glad that these operations are out of the way, because now we can get back to building her up again.'

When his wife had to go into hospital for a hip replacement, Max was angry at how little the hospital staff seemed to understand about dementia, particularly when he found his wife wandering in the hospital car park in bare feet wearing only her nightie.

> 'The hospital system is not trained to deal with people with dementia, and so when people with dementia go into hospital for other health reasons they are not properly looked after because the staff think they're being difficult. They are allowed just to wander, which may be fine most of the time, but can be terribly worrying for relatives.'

One study has suggested that as few as one in five people with dementia have had a proper diagnosis of dementia before being admitted into hospital, and their arrival at the hospital is usually through the doors of the Accident & Emergency department. A worrying 42 per cent of all unplanned admissions are people over the age of 80 with dementia, driven into hospital by a crisis. These are statistics that sound familiar to Patrick, a cardiovascular consultant who trained in geriatric medicine. He believes that patients with dementia should be turned around as quickly as possible when they come into hospital, to return them to familiar surroundings.

'They don't like the confusion. People suffering mild dementia can go completely loopy if taken out of their environment, especially after surgery. And anything that requires an anaesthetic can turn someone with mild dementia into someone who can no longer function and who requires permanent care.'

The manager of one dementia-only care home complains that hospital staff don't really understand dementia, and insists that people with dementia should be in secure wards and looked after by fully trained dementia nurses.

'When our residents go into hospital we always provide the ward staff with a "This is me" leaflet, which states their condition, their needs, their habits and their likes and dislikes. Even though it

> clearly states they have dementia, we often receive phone calls asking us what is wrong with them! We're finding that a lot of hospital staff are now being sent on dementia-related training and they really don't have a clue – which isn't surprising, judging by our experiences with local hospitals.'

When someone with dementia is pushed into the hospital system, they may find themselves grouped with patients who have serious mental-health problems. When the demands of caring at home became too much for Simon's mother, his father had to be 'sectioned' – detained for medical assessment under the Mental Health Act. Simon was going to visit every weekend and found that his father was being moved from one 'awful' place to another.

> 'In the early stages they put him in a hospital ward where there were a lot of people with really terrible mental problems. There were people there who were totally off the scale, going crazy and screaming all day. Dad definitely knew what was going on, and all that was making it so much worse for him. That's not how he should have been treated.'

According to national guidelines, antipsychotic drugs should be given to people with dementia only in cases of severe distress or immediate risk of harm. When a national audit looked at case notes of patients with dementia who had been given antipsychotic drugs in hospital, it noted as 'a matter for concern' that 18 per cent of the case notes recorded no reason for administering the drugs. Nearly two-thirds of the case notes audited gave agitation/anxiety or aggression as the justification. The audit team commented that, in the absence of any evidence that non-drug approaches had been tried before resorting to drugs, 'it is not possible to state whether these prescriptions meet NICE guidelines'. In 8 per cent of cases, antipsychotic drugs were given to patients either to control 'disturbance' (through, for example, noise or wandering) or to facilitate investigations or treatment. In the words of the audit report:

> *'Although information is limited, these reasons appear to relate more to the needs of the hospital as an organisation, rather than those of the person with dementia.'*

Government figures show that between a quarter and a third of all hospital beds are occupied by people with dementia, and patients with dementia will usually spend longer in hospital than people without dementia who are being treated for the same condition. That does not lead to good outcomes, according to an expert on geriatric care, who feels that funds should be diverted from keeping these people in hospital towards alternative services in the community.

'The longer they stay in hospital, the higher the risk of pressure sores, falls and incontinence, and they are more likely to be prescribed antipsychotic

medicines. With that scenario it's hardly surprising that, whereas two-thirds of people go into hospital from their own homes, only approximately a third return home. Most will be going into care homes.'

This is something that concerns people in the adult social-care field, who feel that professionals who assess people with dementia when they are in hospital are more likely to conclude that they are incapable of looking after themselves at home.

'When they're in a difficult environment that is not familiar, they will seem more confused than ever – and they will have been ill as well – so it will probably look like they won't be able to cope at home, and people will start looking for a care home for them.'

A prominent voice in adult social care insists that when people with dementia are discharged from hospital and return to their familiar environment, there is a marked improvement in their cognition and far less confusion. He argues that fairness demands that they should be allowed to carry on at home with support to see if they can cope before it is assumed that they will need a care home.

'It's very hard to change culturally, because consultants and doctors only see people in those hospital beds, and they genuinely think that a care home is the best solution. But nobody looks at their best in an acute hospital bed.'

a story of timing

'I wish I'd moved Mum in with us earlier and been more forceful two years ago, instead of letting her tell me that she was all right. She wouldn't admit it, but I knew she was very lonely.'

David's mother had lived for years in a little village with a good group of friends and a strong community. The village was very poorly served by public transport, and she knew that she would have to stop driving at some stage, so she took the precaution of moving to a nearby town with a decent railway service. This gave her the independence to travel and see her son when she chose, but it also meant she was leaving her supportive network of friends. Early signs of memory problems soon began to appear, which seemed to sap her self-confidence, and her apparent coldness towards her old friends meant that her contact with them dried up very quickly.

'It took me a few years to find out, but she wasn't accepting invitations to go out to see people because of a couple of bad experiences at friends' houses, when she had failed to recognise people she knew.'

David's plan had been to move her in with him and his wife while she was still independent enough to get to know the area and develop new friendships.

> 'I thought at that stage she'd be able to start having a normal life here much more quickly. But actually, by the time we did move her, I think we were about two years too late. If I'd managed to move her sooner, I think her quality of life would be much better right now.'

David feels that his mother would still have had the ability and confidence to explore a bit and would have been happy to walk to the shops and buy a newspaper. He believes that would have made the transition easier for her and, with hindsight, he wishes that he had been more insistent.

> 'But I accept there has to be a balance. If she's saying, "No, I don't want to move", then the only way of being "insistent" is to turn into a bully, and insist that she comes to live with us. Well, where's the joy in that?'

Two other factors contributed to the delay. Firstly, the community psychiatric nurse who was visiting her at home argued against the move. Although she accepted that David's mother was losing her cognitive skills, and would be completely at a loss if she was dropped into the middle of a huge supermarket, she was still of the opinion that his mother was perfectly happy living on her own in her own home and was capable of functioning independently within her own sphere. Secondly, when David did decide that it was time to make the move and began to persuade his mother it was the best course of action, he wanted her to have a self-contained space in his house, paid for by the sale of her own house (he and his siblings calculated that the overall cost would still be less than the expense of paying for her to go into a care home). The structural changes to convert the spare room and bathroom into a granny flat turned out to be more complex than anticipated, and the constraints of planning permission slowed things down further.

> **'So by the time she got here, she had already lost the ability to go out on her own, because she was starting to get lost at home on a regular basis. So now – this is a harsh word, and it's emotional for me – I sometimes think that I've imprisoned my mother, because she is now incapable of going out without one of us to help her.'**

Even with those self-critical regrets, David is convinced that his mother's quality of life has stabilised and she is no longer as lonely as she was. Although he knows that most people are not in a position where they could invite someone with dementia into their home life, and he has no illusions about the demands that are to come, he is still happy that it is the right solution for them.

> **'I suppose my dream is to have Mum die here. She has always loathed the idea of going into a home. It has always been a particular fear with her, because she had a miserable time in institutions when she**

was growing up. That's why I made the decision to have her come and live with us. She gave us a bloody good childhood, and was a very loving mother, so it just feels the right thing to do. But I'm also aware that there may be a time when going into a care home could be the best thing for her – we shall have to see.'

care homes

Should a person with dementia be at home, surrounded by things they know? Or do they need professional full-time care? For children looking after a parent, there may be the extra option of moving the person with dementia into their home. One of the most harrowing questions that carers will face is where their loved ones with dementia should be cared for. The answer should be simple: they should be where they can get the best care for the current stage of the disease. However, the simplicity of that answer is fogged by practical limitations, by expectations and – worst of all – by guilt.

However well supported the main carer may be, there is likely to be a point in the timeline of people with dementia when the demands of care become too difficult to achieve at home. Even with professional help coming into the family home, the situation can deteriorate to the extent that things could be done better elsewhere – whether that is because of carer exhaustion, accelerated decline in the person with dementia or a combination of both of these factors.

It's a huge change that often brings its own debilitating undercurrent of guilt. Even though almost everyone will tell you that you've done the right thing, that you have done all you can, you will still feel that you could have done more and that you should have done more.

There are two types of guilt: healthy guilt and its poisonous opposite number, unhealthy guilt. Healthy guilt is your conscience telling you that you should have done something differently, so that you can change your behaviour. Its unhelpful counterpart – unhealthy and inappropriate guilt – has no such rational basis, but is a very common and understandable reaction to taking a very difficult decision.

'Even now, to this day, I feel guilty. Having coped for a number of months, I said to the hospital people, "I wish I could get her into a home" ... and that's the last thing old people want to hear. If I heard my son say, "We want to get you in a home, Dad," I'd feel terrible! But I was trying to get her into full-time care ... Maybe I should have looked after her for a little longer ... but the hospital agreed that she needed 24-hour care.'

Experts suggest that the best way to stop this destructive feeling of guilt is to tackle it head on. Challenge those inner voices out loud, because hearing it said aloud really can expose the faulty logic behind the guilt. If you are uncomfortable talking to yourself, use a trusted friend as a sounding board.

Was there really more that you could have done? Won't there actually be better full-time care somewhere where the staff are trained and come on fresh at each shift change? Won't this change mean that you can concentrate with fresh energy on befriending and soothing and comforting the person with dementia?

When the family carer is heavily involved in the day-to-day delivery of care, it is often an outsider who sees that it may be time to think differently, and who has the objectivity required to make that judgement. For Alex, that outsider was the GP, who had taken a close interest in his mother's decline, and would call in to visit her occasionally. Alex was concerned at his mother's unwillingness to eat, her depression and her constant talk of dying, and he was frightened that she was going to slowly die of starvation.

'We walked back to his car after he had seen Mum, and he said, "You're right, we have to get her into a care home right now." I asked what had changed, and he said, "You and the carers are not managing this: she really needs professional care from nurses. She needs to be somewhere with a structure and a rhythm where someone else is calling the shots." And he was clear that it couldn't happen at home.'

That is not easy to hear. There's an instinctive feeling deep inside most family carers that a care home should be the very last resort. Caring for a spouse through thick and thin is seen as part of the deal – '... in sickness and in health, to love and to cherish, till death us do part'. Caring for an unwell parent can be regarded as one of the duties of a loving son or daughter, repaying the love that they received in their childhood. But the caring doesn't stop if you have to enlist outside help and move the person with dementia into a care home: it just becomes shared.

Either way, as Charlotte remembers, it's a horrible feeling when you realise that the situation is getting out of control, and that you are going to have to take that decision to change the way care is given. Her mother was seen more and more often by neighbours wandering in the road, and she was even brought home a few times by concerned strangers, which made Charlotte terribly distressed.

> **'It's the moment that everybody dreads, after that initial shock when you are told that your mum does have dementia. You hope that they can just keep managing on their own, but it was all falling apart at home. I was going down as often as I could, and I knew it wouldn't work having her to live with us.'**

Most people imagine that putting someone with dementia into a care home will mean that they stay there until the end, but it need not be such a final step. Gillian found the middle stages of her husband's dementia the hardest to deal with, and when she could cope no more she agonised over the thought of putting him in a home.

> 'But his consultant said to me, when I was in floods of tears, that putting him in a care home needn't be for ever. "You can have him home again whenever you're ready – and you will find that the later stages, when he has lost his aggression and mobility, are much easier to manage." So that's what I did.'

Clare remembers talking about her father to a specialist in dementia care who listened to her story and then asked if she had heard of 'the tipping point', the stage where the person with dementia needs constant trained care.

> 'During this conversation, I actually started to cry because I felt I had reached that stage. And she said, "I think you're way past the tipping point. This is now really quite urgent." I started to feel that I was in danger of neglect, of doing harm because I was trying so hard to keep him in his own home. I knew that he wouldn't mix well in an institution, and that it would be so against everything that he would have wanted, and against everything that I had tacitly agreed with him. It was all done out of love, but perhaps I wasn't doing him a service.'

Charlotte also felt terribly reluctant to move her mother out of her home where everything was familiar and where she had lived for years. She looked into how she might use modern technology to keep an eye on her mother, even considering having pressure sensors installed in doorways to alert a call centre if she tried to leave the house. But in the end she decided that the only choice was to move her to a care home closer to where she and her family were living.

> **'I must have looked at 20 or 30 homes, but what I was trying to do was find the perfect one. Well, there probably isn't a perfect home, you just have to take the best you can get. But seeing some of them made me weep – just reading the social-services reports on some made me weep, so I didn't bother going to see those ones. Others made me despair just talking to staff on the phone.'**

One bad experience can show just how genuinely traumatic it can be when you get it wrong. When her mother declined and became quite confused, Marie was pressed by officials to put her into care. Unable to move her in with the family, she quickly found somewhere near her mother's home that was furnished in a sympathetic way and seemed welcoming. Even so, she felt deep inside that the time was just not right, and was in tears as she listened to the manager assuring her that everything would be fine.

> **'I felt treacherous. I remember going for a walk, thinking it was the worst moment of my life, actually to be putting my mother in a home. Then after two hours I went back, and there was my mother and the social worker both sat there with**

> faces like thunder. They said she wouldn't even have a cup of tea. The manager was worried that Mum was going to hyperventilate and go into crisis. "I can't have her in here!" he told me. It felt almost like they were trying to force her in there, like an animal – and she knew! She said she was never going in there again!'

If you're not familiar with care homes, many can seem quite rigid and institutionalised at first glance, but a huge variety of styles and regimes are on offer in most areas. Giving yourself the time to look at as many options as possible is essential, advises Clare, so that you're not rushed into making a decision under pressure if there is a sudden decline in the health of the person with dementia.

> 'The care homes are all so different. Some are huge homes with a dementia wing; some are really flash, with big double bedrooms and en-suite bathrooms; and some are more like houses, so they feel much more homely and intimate. Looking at all these different places over a series of weekends really helped in making the decisions for Dad. But after a day of looking at different places, you'll probably have the most horrendous headache.'

There is no real substitute for going to see the homes yourself. Visiting a number of homes will help you focus on the details of what sort of atmosphere you are looking for. Whatever they look like on paper or on a website, the reality may be quite different when you walk in and look around.

Pester people for recommendations in your area. Ask all the professionals you come into contact with, including the GP, social services, memory clinic and NHS mental-health team, and talk to anyone you know in a similar position. Personal recommendations can be very valuable – although those giving advice may be judging care homes with very different priorities in mind. Online directories have ratings systems, although they may not tally with your personal ratings.

Some families may feel that the level of comfort will be the most important consideration for their loved one to relax and feel at home. Others will concentrate on the management style or ethos of the home. Above all, make time to meet the manager, because the manager's leadership style and beliefs will lay the foundation for how the home is run.

'Sit down and talk to the manager about your loved one, what stage they are at, what sort of care you are looking for – and you may have very specific questions about your situation. We liked the homes where we were greeted by the manager who would show us round and talk to us about the team – we would always ask how long they had been working together. There are a lot of new homes popping up, but we wanted a team that had been together for a decent amount of time and worked well together, more like a little family – and that's what attracted us to the home where Dad is.'

At other homes Clare visited, she was whisked around by somebody who was looking quite stressed, and who pointed at rooms and ran through an over-rehearsed patter before showing her out again. She was given no chance to sit down and take it in slowly or discuss the principles and practice of care. Clare found that some places seemed to have little interest in engaging with the residents or offering them stimulating activities.

Charlotte was also keen that her mother would be kept active if she had to be placed in a care home, and always asked how the residents in each home were encouraged to fill the day, what they could do to break the monotony.

> 'Mum was used to going into town, visiting her friends or pottering about – what would she do in a home? I asked at this one place and was told they did lots of different things. "I was trying to teach this woman how to crochet," the person told me, "and I don't know why I bothered because she just couldn't get it!" So I realised that there are people working with dementia patients who just don't understand the first thing about dementia. If they've done crochet all their life, then you let them carry on, but you wouldn't expect them to learn something new – it's staggering really ...'

She became used to quizzing staff and managers about their approaches to people with dementia, and often discovered what their real attitudes were by simply watching them in action and listening.

'You could tell straightaway in a home whether the front-line workers had an interest in the lives of the people, or whether they just wanted to institutionalise them. In one home, there was a man sitting looking at a book, and this carer said very dismissively, "Oh, you look at that same book all day long." And I immediately thought, "Well, we won't be coming here again!"'

As you visit different homes, and become accustomed to the features most homes have in common, you will probably find yourself starting to develop a blueprint of the qualities that you are really looking for in a care home. The questions will take shape in your head and your instincts will sometimes give you the answers very quickly. Is this somewhere Dad would be happy? Will they treat him with dignity? Can I imagine visiting him here? Those were the concerns for Gail as she tried to find somewhere for her father.

'Something we discovered as we were looking at these places was that it didn't matter how flash a home was, it was all about how the staff were interacting with the patients, and how the patients seemed when you were there. I remember going to this one home, which was beautiful and had really fantastic facilities, but there were just a lot of people sitting in chairs looking unhappy and staring into space. And we thought that's not somewhere that we want him to be.'

It may take a number of visits and a good deal of determination but it is certainly possible to find good homes that really deserve the title of 'care' homes. So many variables in taste and expectation are involved that nobody else can predict which home you might choose, so keep looking. The more homes you visit, the more you will probably find that you are discovering what really matters to you and your loved one. Dee was keen to find somewhere for her husband where the staff would be able to recognise that, even with dementia, he was still a real person whose patterns of behaviour were part of his character and whose simple habits could and should be accommodated without disruption.

> 'We looked very carefully at a lot of homes and grilled people on how they dealt with dementia. I started to relax in the home we eventually chose when the manager was telling us about a new resident who was becoming very distressed, getting up at 5am and acting aggressively. "If somebody is getting upset," he said, "the philosophy is to try to look at what is upsetting them. We contacted the family, and found that he usually got up early, made himself a piece of toast and wandered round the garden for a few hours. So we told the night staff to allow him into the kitchen to make toast, and the door is unlocked to let him into the garden." And of course that was the end of that particular behavioural problem.'

You may feel totally exhausted in your search for the right home, both in physical terms as you visit all the homes on your list of 'possibles', and in emotional terms as you prepare to take the big step of handing over your loved one to professionals. Most families find this a very distressing time, but there will be real comfort when you do discover a place that lives up to your expectations with staff who have been properly trained so that you can trust them to give appropriate care with the warmth and professionalism you would expect.

> 'The relief was knowing that he would be safe and secure and properly looked after when he was in the home, knowing that it was a home we had chosen, and knowing that we all believed that it was the best possible place for him to be.'

It may take as many as 20 or 30 visits to find somewhere suitable, as Charlotte found, but it really is worth persevering until you track down somewhere that gives you confidence, somewhere that you will be prepared to visit without reluctance so that you can see your loved one through this new phase.

> 'In the end we found this home which we thought was lovely. There was no staffroom, and all the staff on breaks would sit down with the residents and interact with them, even eating their meals with them. The residents seemed happy and it was quite a small home too, which we liked, and

> it was dementia-only. We found that in some of the bigger homes the dementia patients were shut off in a wing to the side, and we didn't want him to feel more locked-in than he needed to be. We wanted somewhere friendly, and we were so impressed with the attitude of the staff – and it was hundreds of pounds cheaper than the big flash place we had seen!'

Even when you have chosen a care home you like, nobody who has been through putting a parent or spouse into care will ever pretend that the actual move is easy. As Carrie remembers, the day when the move had to be made was a turbulent affair.

> 'That day was fairly terrible. While my daughter and a carer were downstairs trying to keep my mother occupied – she was in tears and saying she wanted to die – I was upstairs ironing name tapes on to all her clothes.'

Carrie describes the experience as frantic and bewildering after a sudden decline in her mother's cognitive abilities took the whole family by surprise.

> 'Because I didn't realise this was coming so fast, I hadn't organised things at all. But a friend had these iron-on labels, and I spent hours putting them on. I had to go through all my mother's clothes, because they can't wash clothes

separately and care for special fabrics in these homes. Then I had to buy her a whole load of cotton clothes, which wouldn't get ruined in the wash, and do the name tape thing again.'

For Barbara's mother, the care home started as a temporary fix after she collapsed at home, but she found that being there for a week with good care dissolved her prejudice against being 'put in a home'.

'That first time, I just told her, "This is where you're going to stay." She needed a break, my brother and his wife needed a break, and I needed a break. Mum took three or four days to recover and be herself again because she was having regular meals and taking her pills, but she quite enjoyed it in the end.'

When she came out after a week, she was happy to go home, but she wasn't looking after herself well. Barbara describes it as 'the old roller coaster' – getting worse, getting better, getting worse again – and within four weeks she had another crisis.

'I rang up the care home again, and they said bring her round, so she went in for another week. We probably did that about three or four times, and then there was a day when Mum said she actually felt safer in that environment than she did in her own home – so she stays there now.'

the care-home story

As awareness of dementia grows in Britain, there's a culture of change in care homes. New establishments are opening with a clear mission as to how to give the best care to people who are in the grip of dementia ... so we asked one care home to describe their approach.

Before new residents arrive at the home, the families are asked to write a brief history of who they are and their life before dementia, including their jobs, their hobbies and any interests that could still give them pleasure or help them find a sense of purpose in their day.

> 'We have one lady who used to clean brass one day a week, so we encourage her to continue doing that. We found some brass and a cloth for her to use, and it totally relaxes her. And there's another gentleman who loved gardening, so we encourage him to go out into the garden with a watering can.'

Knowing people's backgrounds is helpful when the home is planning activities to vary the daily routines. They may include anything from pure entertainment, such as an Elvis impersonator, to quieter and more contemplative activities, such as a petting zoo, where the residents can spend some time gently stroking the small animals that are brought in.

The first days in an unfamiliar environment can be disconcerting for new residents, even when they may appear to be spending more time in their private zone, remote from their surroundings. Families are encouraged to bring in familiar personal items for the bedrooms – photos, ornaments, perhaps even a favourite chair – to make the room more individual and comforting for the person with dementia.

> **'There needs to be a settling-in period when a new client arrives. We recommend the family give them time to adjust by not visiting for three days up to a week. It really depends on the individual but we will speak daily with the family to provide updates and advise when the time is right for a first visit.'**

Most of the new entrants have been cared for either in their own homes or with family, and are moving into care because they need full-time attention or because the family carer can no longer cope with the stresses. But some people with dementia come to the home after spending time at other institutions, and sometimes their families are moving them in desperation at the low standards of care in other homes that either couldn't care or didn't care.

> **'A lady has just joined us after two bad experiences elsewhere. When I went to fetch her, she was sitting alone in a chair with her head hanging to one side with dribble down her front. She was practically blind and had apparently been left there like that for hours drugged up.'**

Staff took extra care to walk this lady around the home for the first few days, so that she could get used to the layout and the people. They also took her off the medication that had been sedating her.

'We don't believe in giving our clients antipsychotic drugs. Everyone has their own personality and we embrace that. This is something to watch out for when looking at various homes.'

So how would the staff of one care home advise a family to find a good home that is fit for their loved one? Their recommendation is that you use the website of the Care Quality Commission (www.cqc.org.uk), which lists thousands of care homes throughout Britain, including the best homes in each area. The site gives access to the CQC inspectors' reports together with inspection dates, and is a good resource to help you in your search.

'When you find a home you like, speak to the families of other residents there. A good care home should never require an appointment to visit and the office door should always be open to residents and families.'

Echoing widespread concerns about the quality and training of the staff you will find in the care homes, they recommend that you should try to find an established team who have been working together for a decent period of time. Since good communication skills are vital, they are critical of homes that employ too many foreign staff who may struggle to make themselves understood.

> 'We are very popular in the area because of our high rating and we have no plans to expand. A lot of homes in the area are constantly expanding because of increased demand, and that means they lose the personal touch. A person who is suffering from dementia needs constant mental stimulation and not everywhere is capable of providing this.'

As they drift in and out of confused memories, the mood of each resident is constantly changing. Knowing how short their concentration spans can be, staff focus on getting to know the individual and thinking up ways to arouse their interest and stimulate interplay with others.

> 'There are still those short periods when they mentally come back and these moments are so precious. As we don't have a separate staffroom, the staff and residents mix throughout the day and there is constant interaction. We keep to a routine for meals but there are no set bedtimes and you get to know the habits of each client.'

Some families just can't cope with visiting, so the staff try to ensure that nobody is left out, even buying little presents for them to open on Christmas Day, with everyone making an effort to get dressed up. In the homes where 'care' is at the heart of their thinking, there can be real warmth in the staff's efforts to ensure that each day is rewarding for the residents.

> 'We all get attached and very upset when our residents die. We can't leave them at the end and have often stayed with them through the night. Sometimes we can seem to be more upset than their families, because a lot of their grieving is done earlier with this illness.'

When the person with dementia does die, the staff take great pains never to put pressure on the families to clear their loved one's bedroom.

> 'Families will come and see us afterwards. It can be hard for them to let go. There are some who keep coming back to have dinner and cups of tea with us – we would never turn them away.'

visiting on their terms

So you've moved into the next stage of caring, where professionals will take charge of the everyday care of your loved one, and you can allow yourself to be transformed from full-time carer to top-class visitor and companion.

Care homes will often suggest that you don't visit for the first week or so, to allow the person with dementia to settle in and become used to the new routines and facilities. This is naturally very upsetting for many relatives. It can seem like you are abandoning your loved one. Try to think of it as time for you to regroup, catch up on rest and prepare to give of your best in this new phase.

> 'After Mum first went into the hospice, Dad went home and slept through for eighteen hours. He hadn't realised how shattered he was, not just emotionally drained, but completely physically exhausted.'

You may need renewed strength for your first visit, as seeing your loved one in a different setting can be tough. The best homes will make a real effort to create a personal space for each individual, and will work hard to integrate newcomers and make them feel at home, as Fiona found when her father moved to a nearby care home.

> 'He actually seemed to settle in quite quickly ... and the home was fantastic. We hung some of his pictures around the home, and he was told that it was an art exhibition, so he loved that. He also plays the piano and within a few days he was playing in the afternoon for the residents, which they all loved – and it cheered the staff too.'

Even where extraordinary care, such as this, has been taken, subsequent visits can still take you by surprise and shatter the peaceful view that all is now well, as Fiona found on her next visit to her father.

> 'I found him up in his room, which we had made really nice; but he had taken all the paintings down off the walls and he was trying to hide them because he was worried that people would steal them. He just looked so different. He asked me when his mum was coming, and when I explained that she couldn't come today he just burst into tears and sobbed and sobbed, saying he didn't understand what was going on.'

Visiting the person you love in a care home is never going to be easy. The best advice is that you visit when you are feeling primed for a challenge, choosing a time that is good for you and, of course, that fits in with the routine at the home.

> 'I usually see her once or twice a week. I have to go when I'm feeling upbeat. I've found now that I can walk to this place, which is brilliant. I get there having had a really good walk, and I take my lead from her. She's always in the main room when I arrive, and she usually looks at me and she beams ...'

In most homes, residents lead a collective existence. They will spend the largest part of their day in the main room and this means that you may encounter people at all sorts of stages of dementia during your visit, which can be disconcerting – so it's wise to be ready for anything.

> 'All these people are so different from each other in the way their dementia manifests itself. There was one chap who just sat and slightly rocked all the time. Another woman had her handbag with her and her coat on all the time because she was "Just going ...", always "Just going ...". When I first went there, I thought she was a visitor because she seemed quite lucid. She'd say, "Right, I'll be off now, so I'll see you later on," and I'd say goodbye to her. And then a few minutes later she'd appear again and say, "Well, I'll be off now," and so it went on.'

Some people are good visitors, and some are not. Some feel awkward, as though they need reassurance from the person they're visiting that it's worth them being there – and that reassurance does not always come. It really does pay dividends if you can plan something to do that might have some meaning for the person you're visiting.

> 'I've seen so many visitors who just sit there looking at their watches, next to their supposed loved ones, not touching them, not interacting at all. And they say, "Well, it's been lovely to see you," and their loved one just stares at the floor, and they kiss them and their loved one stares at the same floor, and then they go. End of visit.'

If you go to visit out of duty and are cowed by the circumstances – the room, the wallpaper, the other relatives, the other residents, or just the misery of the whole situation – then the visit is going to be tough for you and your loved one. Of course, it's easier to think that they're as nutty as a fruitcake and that nothing you do will make any difference. But your visit really can help, if only you communicate the love that brought you through the traffic and the deadlines.

'When my father took me to see his uncle who had dementia, I was hopeless. I just stood there open-mouthed and cried to see how this lovely man had just shrivelled. My father sat with him, talked with him, laughed with him and sympathised with him – I'm sure he warmed his soul, and it taught me so much about how to visit, and how to give that sense of love.'

Several carers have suggested that visits should be approached like any other important project – prepare before the visit and review the results. What went well? What failed? What flustered you, and how can you come to grips with it differently next time? A trick that really helped Jim to develop a good visiting plan was keeping a brief diary note of each visit.

'When Dad first went into care, I stayed with him for hours and I had really quite a bad time. So after each visit, I rated how well it had gone,

giving it a mark out of ten, and then I described what we did and how I felt he was and what I did with him that worked. It helped me get a structure in place, and helped me engage with what was happening. It wasn't a diary of my feelings, it was a grading of the quality of time that we had had together.'

Jim's diary was not about the progress of the dementia and how it was affecting his father. It focused on how successful the interaction between the two of them had been at each visit.

'It helps me be a little detached about it all, as well, rather than saying how heartbreaking it is to see him like this – that is not what it's about.'

Making the brief entries and giving each visit marks out of 10 forced Jim to think about the visit, and to evaluate which activities or conversations his father seemed to enjoy most. And since helping his father feel good also gave Jim great pleasure, it encouraged him to visit more often and to build on the successes.

'The other way this grading in the diary helped me was that I might come back feeling down and disappointed after what felt like a really awful visit, and I would start to write "2 out of 10". But I could look back in the diary and see another visit that I had graded "2 out of 10" and think, "Oh, this visit wasn't as bad as that one! That was a really, really awful visit!" So I ended up grading it as "4 out of 10". It helped me to gauge how my visits were going, and how well he was doing.'

Some families rarely visit, according to the manager of one care home, perhaps because they never had a close relationship with their parents. Other families are much closer and visit whenever they can, and at least every weekend.

'We find that visits tend to diminish as the dementia gets worse. The families feel their loved ones are safe and it's hard for them to see the state they have reached. It becomes like somebody else in their dad's body and it's not good for him to see them upset.'

If you can think of an interest or passion that reaches deep into the heart and soul of someone with dementia, then that may well be the place to start when you're considering how to focus a visit on giving pleasure and communicating love and warmth. It may be a hobby or a sport or the holiday of a lifetime; or it might be something much simpler and more general. Often the pursuit or passion that arouses most interest is one that dates back to an earlier time.

Fran's mother had always loved babies and little children, and when she catches sight of a baby now, Fran feels as though her real mother comes to the surface.

'In the first home there was this great-grandchild who would come in and my mother loved seeing him. So I bought a lovely coffee-table book of professional black-and-white photographs of babies and very small children. We would look at that together for half an hour, just turning the pages, looking at their eyes, touching their noses ... and she'd go somewhere inside herself, somewhere happy. It was brilliant.'

Photographs can be generally very effective in conjuring up good thoughts and feelings, if they're chosen carefully. Since the dementia tends to obliterate more recent memories as it progresses, but leaves earlier memories untouched, carers find that older photographs create a better atmosphere for gentle reflection. They help the person with dementia make contact with old and pleasant memories.

'I took in photographs of her and her family from when she was a child, much better than recent ones of my family when the children were young. With those old black-and-white pics, we could sit for hours, talking and just looking ...'

When Emma visited her mother in the home after work, she would take in her favourite biscuits and little cakes to share with some of the other residents. She soon found herself slipping into a sort of maternal role as they clustered around her.

'I used to tell Mum and a friend stories every evening. The irony is that they were the stories she used to tell me, and I was telling them back to her. She loved listening to the stories, and the residential home was really thankful because it was like having another pair of hands for them. All the little ladies used to come round eventually, and I'd be sitting there telling them these stories until they all went to bed.'

In trying to find an activity that her mother would enjoy, Kath started to take in her guitar when she visited the care home. She saw other residents smiling and taking an interest, noticed a few feet tapping here and there, and gradually some of them would join in and sing the old songs.

'I've learnt some songs that I never thought I would learn – "We'll Meet Again', 'Ain't She Sweet' – some of my mum's old favourites that I had never played on the guitar. She would always sit and listen; sometimes she would join in and sometimes she wouldn't.'

Wondering if her concentration on getting the chords right on the guitar might be getting in the way, Kath left her guitar at home on the next visit. When she held her mother's hand and started to sing, her mother's face relaxed and she quickly joined in, and Kath could feel the electricity of creating that shared moment together. With nods and smiles of recognition, a handful of the other residents soon picked up the song, and Kath sensed a warmth spreading between them as the old songs floated them back to gentler times.

Whatever ingenious ideas you come up with, they won't work for ever. You are likely to discover that each of them has a shelf life, a period when they will succeed in giving pleasure and channel warm feelings. Then you will have to move on and find something new.

'Now I find that we can't do the photographs any more. She just looks at them and says, "Right, where shall we go?" which means, "Enough!"'

Not everybody will feel able or willing to visit a friend or relative with dementia, even when that person is still living at home. And it is more unsettling when he or she has moved into the final stage, and is being looked after in a care home. It's easy to feel that these people are wrong not to visit, but to some older people, seeing an old friend or a sibling in obvious distress can be an uncomfortable and harrowing reminder of how close their own end may be.

'All the people who were in my mother's life have dropped away now. Her brother has said to me he doesn't think it's a good idea for him to go and visit. He always asks how she is doing. I don't tell him she's forgotten who he is, but I might say she's really forgotten everybody, but she doesn't ask after anyone now, and he's not doing a bad thing by not going.'

And some visits really may be awful – when nothing you say sounds right, or when your loved one is just agitated or distant. Visits like this are upsetting for all concerned, and unhelpful for the person with dementia. There may be other worries gnawing at you, making you feel you should be somewhere else. There may also be days when everything just seems grey and hopeless.

> 'Sometimes I would go there and he would be really, really down and crying and talking of dying. And I wouldn't know what to do except say things like "I'm glad I'm here with you" or "Yes, I'm sure you feel that way and I can understand that. I can't help you in that, but I can help you by holding your hand." It became exhausting doing that over and over again, because each time he would forget that we had just been through it.'

When your visits are as draining as that, you may have to fall back on a more primitive means of communicating. Where conversation may carry with it the fear of ambush, of reaching a verbal cliff edge when the right words are beyond your loved one's reach, try touch. A soothing massage of a hand and the gentle touch of a friend or relative can give enormous comfort and a feeling of calm reassurance to someone who is struggling to control high levels of internal distress.

> 'What we are doing at the moment, which is working very well, is gently rubbing her hands

with moisturising lotion, all the way up to the elbows. We can usually do that for 40 minutes or so. The touch is so relaxing. You're transmitting love, and they can feel it.'

Focusing on how your interaction feels to the person with dementia may help you make the most of your time together. Anne discovered that she could turn the frustrations of her father's constant repetition into a useful bond between them when it occurred to her that maintaining the conversation between the two of them was more significant than what they talked about. Although at first she worried that it felt 'insulting' or patronising to discuss the same subject, using the same words repeatedly, she realised that if her father got as much pleasure from telling her of old experiences a second time as he had the first time, then repetition was effectively making him twice as contented.

'Once you learn the idea of "going with them" then it's easier. When Dad is completely "off with the fairies" I sit and chat with him for two hours at a stretch, because I feel it matters to talk to him. And the conversation may be repeating the same thing for half of that time – but actually he loves it and it is easier for me, because if I run out of things to say, we can start again! What matters to both of us is that we enjoy an engaged and active conversation together for a few hours.'

The buzzword, or phrase, in discussions about giving the best care is 'person-centred care'. It's a phrase with many definitions, but the core value for the family carer, once you have reached the care-home stage, is the simple idea of giving the person with dementia as much loving attention as he or she is able to absorb. Time will lose its meaning for people in the later stages of dementia, but carers know they have only a limited time to offer that nourishing love.

'He's really forgotten "me", but he gets the feeling that there's love there. So that next time I go in he looks at me and there's warmth in his expression, rather than confusion or blankness. What is important is to make sure that, for the few hours I'm with him, he and I have as good a time as we are able to have. He won't remember it in the same way that I will, but the feelings will stay with him when the memory of what happened has gone. But it's going to stay with me for always.'

USEFUL CONTACTS

When you want comprehensive information on a particular aspect of dementia care, advice on a specific question or somewhere to share your concerns and draw strength from the experiences of others in a similar position, almost all roads lead to the *Alzheimer's Society*. It has many faces: it is the organisation that moves in high lobbying circles, helping government bodies behind the scenes, and it is also the local support worker or helper in Dementia Cafés across Britain. You can tap into their experts' collected wisdom on the internet, through videos on YouTube, podcasts you can download and listen to in the car, or by browsing through their enormous collection of information sheets to get you up to speed on a range of topics. You can also use the services of a local dementia adviser from Alzheimer's Society offices across the country.

The National Dementia Helpline on 0300 222 1122 offers an advice and information service to anyone affected by dementia, including people with dementia, their carers and family members, and medical or social-care professionals. If you prefer to e-mail your question, you will find a form on the Alzheimer's Society website.

'We try and answer any question about dementia, anything at all. So that could be questions about diagnosis, details on how the disease affects the brain, information about benefits or legal rights – right up to the decoration of care homes.'

Everybody who works on the helpline has extensive training, and is backed up by information specialists who can dig out answers to more complex questions, drawing on the database and library resources of the Alzheimer's Society. The helpline doesn't offer specialist legal, financial or medical advice, but aims to give people information in those areas so they can make their own choices.

'A significant number of calls to the helpline are from people concerned about a person in the early stages of dementia – questions about the symptoms, what should people look out for and information about medication. But we also get a lot of calls from people dealing with the middle and later stages, which might be about coping with particular behavioural symptoms, or looking at residential care or end-of-life care.'

Calls to the helpline may be for practical advice, perhaps for the answer to a specific question that is troubling the caller, and most can be answered there and then. However, some callers ask questions that require further research, so the adviser will arrange to call back once the information has been put together. Others are looking for emotional support, and the helpline staff have been trained in the core counselling skills so they know how to listen and be a comforting prop for the callers. The helpline also acts as a useful 'signposting' service, pointing callers to organisations that may be able to offer more detailed help on specific issues.

The Alzheimer's Society also facilitates a non-stop online community for help and advice. This is *Talking Point*, a moderated online forum where people affected by dementia can ask questions and pool experiences. Like any community, it is there for discussions, for help with difficult personal issues and to help you feel supported and part of a network of people who understand and perhaps share your problems and concerns.

The resources available from the Alzheimer's Society cover an enormous number of topics, and other helpful organisations also offer you good advice or support in caring for someone with dementia. The following is a selection of contact points, some offering guidance on specialist subjects (such as driving or finding care homes), while others have a more general focus.

Admiral Nursing DIRECT is a telephone helpline – 0845 257 9406 – provided by Admiral Nurses and supported by the charity Dementia UK. Admiral Nurses are specialist mental-health nurses who provide both practical and emotional support to people affected by dementia.

Adviceguide is a website offering information and factsheets from Citizens Advice on a variety of subjects, including benefits, discrimination and legal issues. www.adviceguide.org.uk

Advicenow is an independent, not-for-profit website that offers helpful information on rights and legal issues for the general public. Law lecturer and broadcaster Marcel Berlins describes it as the liveliest, least stuffy, most accessible and understandable website on legal matters available. www.advicenow.org.uk

The *Age UK advice line* – 0800 169 6565 – provides information about help available through social services, as well as advice on other issues faced by older people. www.ageuk.org.uk

Alzheimer Scotland provides the National Dementia Helpline in Scotland – 0808 808 3000 – as well as local services all over Scotland for people with dementia and their carers. www.alzscot.org

Alzheimer's Disease International describes itself as the global voice on dementia. It offers training and supports national Alzheimer associations, representing them at the World Health Organization. www.alz.co.uk

Alzheimer's Research UK is the leading dementia research charity in the UK, and has put millions of pounds into hundreds of research projects focused on understanding the causes of dementia and finding ways to prevent, treat and ultimately cure dementia. Their website offers leaflets that give clear information about dementia and fundraising packs. www.alzheimersresearchuk.org

Alzheimer's Society provides the National Dementia Helpline for England, Wales and Northern Ireland – 0300 222 1122. It offers information, support, guidance and signposting to other appropriate organisations. www.alzheimers.org.uk

AT Dementia is a charity with Department of Health funding that offers advice and information on how assistive technology can benefit people with dementia. www.atdementia.org.uk

Bettercaring is a search site that offers a database of residential and nursing homes in the UK. All homes registered in the UK are listed, and can be searched by location, facilities, services or cost. www.bettercaring.com

BRACE – 0117 340 4831 – is a Bristol-based registered charity that funds research into Alzheimer's disease and other forms of dementia. www.alzheimers-brace.org

Care UK – 0333 321 8305 – is a major independent provider of health and social-care services for people living with dementia. www.careuk.com

Carers Direct – 0808 802 0202 – is part of the NHS, and offers comprehensive information, advice and support for carers. www.nhs.uk/carersdirect

Carers Trust is a charity formed by the merger of Crossroads Care and the Princess Royal Trust for Carers, and aims to make advice and practical support available to carers across the UK. www.carers.org

Carers UK is a charity that provides information and advice about caring as well as practical and emotional support. www.carersuk.org

Caring with Confidence, funded by the NHS, provides free online training courses to help carers develop their skills at their own speed and improve the care they offer. www.caringwithconfidenceonline.co.uk

Citizens Advice offers free, independent and confidential advice on rights and responsibilities. There are over 3,500 Citizens Advice Bureau locations in England and Wales, and a full telephone advice service is under development. To find your local CAB in England or Wales, go to www.citizens advice.org.uk, in Northern Ireland go to www.citizensadvice. co.uk and in Scotland go to www.cas.org.uk.

The *Care Quality Commission* is the independent regulator of all health and social-care services in England. Its website shows reports on hospitals and care homes to ensure that they meet standards of quality and safety. www.cqc.org.uk

Cognitive Stimulation Therapy is a drug-free alternative to medication for people with mild to moderate dementia. www.cstdementia.com

The *Contented Dementia Trust* is a small charity based in Oxfordshire, which aims to promote the lifelong well-being of people with dementia through the SPECAL method. www.contenteddementiatrust.org

Cruse – 0844 477 9400 – is the UK's largest bereavement charity, and offers one-to-one support, bereavement support groups and a national helpline. www.crusebereavementcare.org.uk

The *Dementia Action Alliance* is a grouping of more than 100 organisations committed to improving the lives of people living with dementia in the UK, as detailed in their National Dementia Declaration. www.dementiaaction.org.uk

DementiaGuide is a Canadian website offering useful general information on dementia to help carers understand and manage dementia symptoms. www.dementiaguide.com

Dementia UK is a charity that supports Admiral Nurses and runs Uniting Carers, a national network of family carers of people with dementia working to raise awareness and understanding of dementia. www.dementiauk.org

Dementia Web – 0845 120 4048 – offers information about dementia and the support and care services available. They also have a 24-hour dementia helpline. www.dementiaweb.org.uk

Disability Rights UK works to support people with any form of disability, and is a good source of fact sheets on, for example, allowances and independent living. www.disabilityrightsuk.org

The *DVLA* (Driver and Vehicle Licensing Agency) is the body responsible for maintaining over 44 million UK driver records, and the Drivers Medical Group within the DVLA is responsible for establishing whether drivers with medical conditions can satisfy the standards required for safe driving. www.dvla.gov.uk

The *Eldercare Team* is an American organisation whose website offers useful information and experiences of caring for elderly people. www.eldercareteam.com

Find Me Good Care, developed and managed by the Social Care Institute for Excellence (see below), helps people make choices about care and support in England. www.findmegoodcare.co.uk

FirstStop Advice is a free service, provided by the Elderly Accommodation Counsel charity, which aims to help older people live independently and comfortably. They offer a national advice line – 0800 377 7070. www.firststopcareadvice.org.uk

The *Frontotemporal Dementia Support Group* (formerly Pick's Disease Support Group) is a source of support and information for people with fronto-temporal dementia and their families. They have a list of regional contact names and numbers on their website. www.ftdsg.org

Healthcare.co.uk provides information to help people get the health care and social care they need, and also features an Independent Living Shop. www.healthcare.co.uk

Healthtalkonline is an online database of personal and patient experiences, and includes videos of interviews with carers of people with dementia. www.healthtalkonline.org/carers/Carers_of_people_with_dementia

Independent Age offers an information and advice service for older people, their families and carers through local offices across the UK, and via an advice line – 0845 262 1863. www.independentage.org

The *Lewy Body Society* provides support and advice to people with dementia with Lewy bodies, their families and carers. You can contact a helpline adviser, in partnership with Parkinson's UK, on 0808 800 0303. www.lewybody.org

The *National Council for Palliative Care* is the umbrella charity for people involved in end-of-life care, and is a source of information and advice, including a guide for carers of people with dementia on helping with pain and distress. www.ncpc.org.uk

Parkinson's UK is the UK's support and research charity for Parkinson's disease, and has a free confidential helpline service – 0808 800 0303. www.parkinsons.org.uk

Patient.co.uk aims to give non-medical people in the UK good and clear evidence-based information about health and disease. www.patient.co.uk

The *Social Care Institute for Excellence* is an independent charity that aims to improve the lives of people who use care services by sharing knowledge about what works. They offer practical guides on social-care issues, a database of good practice and downloadable videos on various topics including dementia. www.scie.org.uk

TheCarer provides information and advice on the challenges facing family carers. www.thecarer.co.uk

The National Careline is a not-for-profit company offering information about care and support for older people, their carers and their families. www.thenationalcareline.org

ACKNOWLEDGEMENTS

This book has been a team effort. To respect their privacy, I am not going to thank by name all the carers we interviewed, but I am so grateful for their contributions. However, I do wish to say a very special thank you to Susanna Abbott, Alex Loxton, Thirza Rockall, Cindy Polemis and Lorna Parker, and most of all to Huw Rowley.

ENDNOTES

DEMENTIA EXPLAINED

27 A major review
National Audit of Dementia Care in General Hospitals (2011). Commissioned and funded by the Healthcare Quality Improvement Partnership, and produced by the Royal College of Psychiatrists' Centre for Quality Improvement. © Royal College of Psychiatrists (2011)

34 A super-champion of memory
Foer, Joshua, US Memory Champion 2006, 'Moonwalking with Einstein'

40 A Swedish study
Karolinska Institutet, Stockholm, *Neurology®* (May 2011)

DIAGNOSIS AND FIRST STEPS

51 recent studies suggest
Alzheimer's Society, *http://www.alzheimers.org.uk/site/scripts/news_article.php?newsID=1463*

54 A recent study by UK researchers
University of Leicester and the National Collaborating Centre for Mental Health, London, examined 30 previous studies involving 15,277 people seen in primary care for cognitive disorders, including 7109 assessed for dementia.

54 a study of London GPs
IPPR report, *Dementia care in London* (March 2011)

CARE AND COMMUNITY

85 A study of older people in the US
Rush University Medical Center, *Journal of the International Neuropsychological Society* (April 2011)

88 a recent study of adults aged between 50 and 68
University of Chicago, *Psychology and Aging* (November 2012)

151 a review of sleep research
Cappuccio FP, D'Elia L, Strazzullo P & Miller MA. Sleep duration and all-cause mortality: a systematic review and meta-analysis of prospective studies. *Sleep* 2010; 33 (5) online. http://www2.warwick.ac.uk/newsandevents/pressreleases/short_sleep_increases/

151 people in one study
Yo-el Ju et al., presented at the American Academy of Neurology (April 2012)
see also R Sterniczuk et al., presented at Neuroscience (October 2012) http://www.abstractsonline.com

151 other research
D Holtzman et al; J. H. Roh, Y. Huang, A. W. Bero, T. Kasten, F. R. Stewart, R. J. Bateman, D. M. Holtzman, *Disruption of the Sleep-Wake Cycle and Diurnal Fluctuation of Beta-Amyloid in Mice with Alzheimer's Disease Pathology*. Sci. Transl. Med. 4, 150ra122 (2012)
see also Kang, J.-E., et al., *Amyloid beta dynamics are regulated by orexin and the sleep-wake cycle, Science Express* (2009)

153 a small-scale study in the Netherlands
Royal Netherlands Academy of Arts and Sciences, *Journal of the American Medical Association* (June 2008)

155 research reveals that the outcome of 20-minute job interviews
Bernieri, Frank; Prickett, Tricia, University of Toledo, Ohio
http://cjonline.com/stories/062501/pro_impressions.shtml
http://chronicle.augusta.com/stories/2001/06/18/bus_313814.shtml

ESSENTIAL TECHNIQUES

167 film study
University of Maryland Medical Center, presented at the Scientific Session of the American College of Cardiology (March 2005)

175 a recent review by public health experts
Boehm, J Boehm; Kubzansky, L, Harvard School of Public Health, *Psychological Bulletin* (April 2012)http://www.hsph.harvard.edu/news/press-releases/positive-emotions-cardiovascular-health/

183 a small-scale study in Sweden
'Can Caregiver Singing Improve Person Transfer Situations in Dementia Care?'
Music and Medicine 4: 237-244 (October 2012) http://dem.sagepub.com/content/10/1/98

195 An American study
Cache County (Utah) Memory Study, *Journal of the American Geriatrics Society* (May 2010)

CARE IN THE LATER STAGES

221 national audit
Report of the National Audit of Dementia Care in General Hospitals (2011).
Commissioned and funded by the Healthcare Quality Improvement Partnership, and produced by the Royal College of Psychiatrists' Centre for Quality Improvement. © Royal College of Psychiatrists (2011)

INDEX

index

index